TOUCHING
PRESENCE

To Ed with much love,

Jessica

Christmas 2014

Tommy's note on the cover photo:

At the top of Mount Pilatus near Lucerne in Switzerland, I witnessed a crow flying from way above us towards the outstretched hand of a man unknown to me. I just happened to capture the photo the moment the bird landed in his hand. For the reason *why* this is the cover photo, read the Preface.

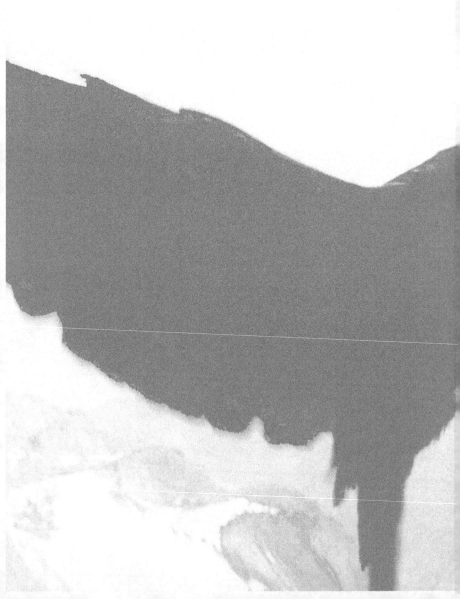

TOUCHING PRESENCE

TOMMY THOMPSON

WITH
RACHEL PRABHAKAR

Ease of Being Publications

Cambridge MA USA
First Edition – 2019

Publisher's Cataloging-In-Publication Data

Thompson, Tommy, 1942–
    Touching presence / Tommy Thompson ; with Rachel
Prabhakar.

    Paperback. 152 p. 5.25in. x 8in. 133mm. x 203mm.
    ISBN 978-1-7334005-0-3
Also issued in electronic e-book format

1. Alexander Technique. I. Title. II. Prabhakar,
Rachel 1970–.

Library of Congress Control Number : 2019911684

First edition published in print in 2019 by

*EaseofBeing
Publications*™

Cambridge MA USA — www.easeofbeing.com

Book and cover design by David Gorman
Photo of cover/title page by Tommy Thompson
Photo in Tommy's biography by Elisabeth Schanda
Photo of Tommy with guitar by Julian Lage
Photo in Rachel's biography by Matilde Barbosa

Contents

Foreword – How this book came to be

I had the privilege of training with Tommy in his Teacher Training Program at the Alexander Technique Center at Cambridge. As a graduation gift, I created a book for Tommy drawn from my notes on his teachings. Other students and teachers immediately said that they wanted copies of the book. In response to those requests, Tommy and I began to work together to prepare a book for more general circulation. We have swapped edits back and forth, and supplemented the original text with additional passages Tommy wrote, with material gathered by me in interviews with Tommy, and with further notes I took during workshops with Tommy. As we neared publication, David Gorman provided invaluable guidance, copy editing, and technical assistance.

For the original book, which forms the backbone of this volume, I started with my handwritten notes jotted down during lectures and discussions from my time in the training, comprising the period of September 2010 through June 2013. I tried to keep as close as possible to Tommy's actual words. The notes are arranged thematically, rather than chronologically. In the training and workshops, themes and topics come up on different days, months, and years. As themes come around over time, Tommy often explores them using different language or from a different perspective, responding to the needs of the audience. Some of that variation comes through here.

I hope that you, the reader, gain as much insight and enjoyment as I have from these discussions.

Presented with deepest love, thanks, and appreciation,

Rachel Prabhakar
Brookline, Massachusetts
July 2019

Introduction

I first met Tommy Thompson in the summer of 1988. I had moved back to Boston and wanted to continue my Alexander teacher training. At the time there were several training courses in the city. I visited two or three programs. When I stepped into Tommy's office, something was different. I felt seen in a way I hadn't been before. It was not alarming or disturbing in any way, it was just quite different from my previous Alexander experiences. Tommy gave me a chair lesson. Since I was a pianist recovering from tendonitis, he put a stool in front of me and had me put my hands on it – like the piano. It was a variation on *Hands On the Back Of The Chair*. Words were said that I didn't completely grasp. But as he worked with his hands I felt a sensation in my own hands that I had never experienced before. It was as if my hands were glowing. That's when he mentioned that was the quality he expected all his trainees to have in their hands when they graduated from his training. Well, that was all I needed to hear. I signed up for his training course soon after.

But there was something else that drew me to Tommy. It was this quality of feeling seen for who I was with complete acceptance. I had already been studying the Alexander Technique for five years, and I had worked with some remarkable teachers. But there was an element of Tommy's teaching that made me feel he was working with ME. Not my body, not a generic person, but ME. I began to address aspects of myself that I had not noticed before. One might say that it took me five years to be ready to notice this and that the other teachers were doing the same. But, honestly, knowing that this is at the core of his teaching, and having witnessed it for over thirty years, I believe it is the single most distinctive element in Tommy's teaching. And it is powerful. It led to my complete recovery from severe tendonitis. That happened when I asked Tommy why, after all this time studying the Technique, I still recognized the sensations of the injury when I spent just a few moments at the piano. He replied that it was all in the *attitude* I took to the piano. That statement led to my discovery of the identity I had created in order to feel worthy of piano playing. It's a long story. But it was Tommy's insight into ME that allowed me to find ME and heal ME via the change and acceptance I was ready to embrace.

Shortly after I graduated from Tommy's training in 1992 I began to assist him in the program. It was a privilege that I still appreciate to this day. Attending the training as a graduate allowed me to experience and re-experience his words, his teaching, his evolution. I was able to hear the words written in this book as though for the first time. And I was able to receive them from a new perspective. Over the last 27 years of teaching I have deepened my understanding of the work, of Tommy's teaching, and of the possibilities for growth in all of us. I always tell my students that I am teaching the Alexander Technique to heal the world by freeing one neck at a time. And since I couldn't reach enough necks I decided to train teachers. This yearning to heal the world, and seeing the Alexander Technique as having a potential role in that, is something I learned from being in Tommy's presence. His ability to see beauty and good in everyone is clear in the words that he has always shared and that he shares here.

This book is a gem. It brings to the Alexander world the language and thinking of a master teacher – one who never tires of exploring the principles of Alexander's discoveries, and who seeks to teach them in the clearest and most honest way possible. The influence of Tommy's time spent with Frank Pierce Jones also shows up here. There is specificity in Tommy's work that manifests at the same time as the open-ended space for new possibilities. And there is a gentleness and support that makes facing ourselves as easy as it can be.

Tommy tells stories in his training course that are profound. They are stories from his life that have clarified his understanding of Alexander's teaching. This book offers the wisdom that has come from living the stories. From *Withholding Definition* as an explanation for Alexander's *Inhibition* to *Seeing the Beauty of the Person* you are teaching, you are about to enter an Alexander world of beauty, gentleness, insight, acceptance and change. I expect you'll enjoy the ride!

Debi Adams
Boston, Massachusetts
July 2019

Preface

On our wedding anniversary in 2001 my wife, Julie, invited me to join her in retreat at Linden Cottage on Linden Farm in the Blue Ridge Mountains of Virginia. The cottage and 200 accompanying acres were owned by her friend Robert Strini, a sculptor who worked out of his barn nearby yet still some distance away from the cottage. For each of the seven previous years, Julie had gone to Linden Cottage for a solitary retreat to write and think in the beautiful, wild natural environment. Her invitation was unexpected, extraordinary, and welcomed. Seeing her on the land allowed me to appreciate in a very special way the magic that Linden Farm held for her. She wrote in her journal, shortly thereafter and prior to receiving the diagnosis of her terminal illness, that our weekend together was the happiest of her life. Afterwards, I asked Bob Strini, who by then had become a close friend, whether I could stay at the cottage each year on the anniversary of our wedding date for the rest of my life to commemorate Julie's and my life together. He has made this available to me.

On one visit, a bird flew into the cottage and was trapped inside. I figured I could simply leave the door to the cottage open and give the bird a means of escape before it got hurt flying around inside the cottage. However, the bird flew into a corner and just sat there, looking at me. I gently clasped both hands around it to bring it outside, and strangely, the bird, a small sparrow, allowed me to do so. I brought it to the front door and released it, tossing it into the air saying aloud, "There... you're free to go."

But the bird flew back into my hand. I repeated, "You're a bird, you belong out here in the sky, you're free to fly." And again I tossed the bird upwards into the air, and again the bird came back. I attempted to repeat the toss towards freedom several more times. Each time the bird fastened its small talons to my fingers and refused to fly. I was consumed with my view of 'bird'. It should be in the sky, not perched on my hand. So I carried the bird, still perched and looking at me, over to a nearby tree. I carefully took the bird's small talons off my hand and placed them on the limb of a tree. "You're a bird," I said quietly, "this is where you belong. You're free to fly." Then I walked back into the cottage.

Standing inside the small living room, my world of definition began to dissolve. To myself I thought, "Wait a minute, I just threw away the opportunity to communicate with a bird, a creature who wanted to stay and explore with me. Who knows why it chose with each toss into the unfettered sky to return and refuse to budge? Yes, I thought, the bird was free to go, to fly back into the sky where it belonged, but the bird was also free to stay in my hand, perched there for some reason known only to it. Freedom knows no real restraints. The bird on some level made a choice to remain with me. I ran back outside to the tree, hoping to find the bird there waiting for my return. Alas! No bird. Because I had defined the limits and boundaries of freedom, I missed an opportunity. As altruistic as my intentions were, they really did not befit the circumstance. Having defined myself and defined the bird, I limited the possibility of some unusual and sacred form of communication. Unawares, I stood before the interrelatedness of life. I stood before Dr. Martin Luther King's "single garment of destiny where we all live together in an interrelated structure of reality." I limited the sacred ordinary.

It is my hope that you, the reader, might inhibit or withhold definition about the boundaries of F. M. Alexander's discoveries. When we keep Alexander's discoveries in mind, we can re-imagine what it means to learn by remembering that the world we live in is a shared world, and you truly find yourself in the other and they in you. You teach what you need to learn. And whatever truth might surface in the exchange between teacher and student comes from mutual self discovery. What is being given to the student is being received by the teacher and the teacher can only give what they receive.

I think now you will understand why I have chosen the cover photograph. I took the picture atop Mount Pilatus in Switzerland. For me, it represents the delicate poise we find as we explore the freedom to choose between the known and unknown, the expected and the unexpected, the habitual and the non-habitual, the sacred and the ordinary.

Tommy Thompson
Belmont, Massachusetts
July 2019

Note: The phrase "sacred ordinary" was coined by my wife, Julie Ince Thompson. She wrote it in the context of a preface to her book of poetry, *UNCLOTHED and Five Other Poems* (Buddenbrooks, Boston, 2005), which was published posthumously to help raise money to endow a scholarship in her name at the Boston Conservatory.

Touching Presence

On the Beauty of the Person

When Julian Lage[1] was in my teacher training program, someone asked me, "What are you really touching when you touch someone?"

Really touching? Put that way, so absolute, I thought, I have no idea. Except that it's not so much a question of *what* you touch, but *who*. I needed to touch someone to answer the question. Julian had his guitar with him that morning. I asked Julian to play his guitar. Then I knew immediately: I was touching his beauty. Any time anyone is exploring who they actually are, there is beauty.

So what do you really touch when you place your hands on someone? You touch the beauty of the person.

The beauty of the person inheres in several parts. One part is in how the person has developed in response to, in interaction with, all the circumstances of their lives. There is inherent beauty in the person being who they are in this moment.

The other part of the beauty of a person lies in their potential. Whoever that person habitually ascribes to being, there is always an endless possibility apart from that known quantity. You can touch the beauty of that infinite potential.

---

1 Julian is a Grammy-nominated jazz guitarist and composer.

* * *

Touch the potential within that person. It's not that you will fix someone by changing their use. Rather, see who shows up in the moment and help them discover it.

* * *

As a teacher, you just want to be surprised. There is so much to a person. And people are so beautifully poised to discover what they have longed for. And that's what you want to see — their poise at their potential moment of discovery. That's the beauty of the person.

* * *

The reason you are there is a deep appreciation of the person undergoing the experience of being themself. Why touch another person if you aren't going to appreciate them?

On Being and Doing

Being vs. doing is a false dichotomy. You are and I am. You can't not be. But you *can* not do.

Trust the fact that if you choose neither to express something nor to repress it, the appropriate response is likely to show up. It will show up because when you withhold definition, you allow in more information. Within you there is a deep well of information seldom tapped, and born not from what you have done and achieved but from who you are in the absence of doing anything — especially that which reinforces your identity as you most readily know yourself.

In early fetal development you are already growing the major life-support organs of support, including the gut and digestive organs, the proto-nervous system, the heart. As you are developing these centers of being which will eventually support your life, your arms, hands, fingers, and your legs, feet, and toes begin to also develop — first as little flippers awaiting their turn to transform into complex, articulated arms and legs capable of doing things and fulfilling desires.

We humans are distinguished from most other creatures by the dexterity of our hands with their opposable thumbs, which along with our marvelous imagination guides these dexterous hands to create tools which in turn bring form to our thoughts and visions. This has allowed us to dominate the planet, until it seems we have found ourselves as a species overemphasizing doing at the expense of being. Our design is the very apple that was eaten, enabling us to tilt the balance between being and doing. Before the doing you is created, the being you is created: in that order. Paramount to what we learn from this teaching is that we tend to define ourselves by what we are capable of doing at the expense of trusting the support of being in relation to something greater than or apart from our desires. We lose a sense of belonging to something apart from what we ourselves create. When life is lived as if out of relation to all that is, we can have a sense of living in isolation. You mistrust your choices because they are all based on past perceptions of what you expect from the future. The balance of life lies in integrating the being and the doing. And that balance is too often compromised by your sense of identity: who you feel you need to be to be you.

If you don't have a sense of your own geography, of yourself relative to what is around you, you end up being what you are doing. Is that really you?

* * *

We seldom walk from a sense of being present where we are. We walk where we are going. We do this because we tend to move in the direction of the focus of our attention. What if we want to walk with a sense of balance, a sense of being present where we are? Try freeing the three necks. Debi Adams, a gifted Alexander teacher who runs a teacher training program at the Boston Conservatory, in Boston, Massachusetts as well as teaching in our training, likes to talk about the three necks of the body: the neck, the wrist, and the ankle. When you free your neck from unnecessary tension, you allow a movement of your head away from the rest of your body, decompressing your spine, allowing it to lengthen. This lengthening has a positive effect on the total pattern of movement throughout your being. It also tends to free up your breathing, and there is nothing like free breathing to make you feel (and be) more in the present.

Likewise, when you free the wrists, you release the hands from holding on to all they have held before. When you free the ankles, you walk from where you are rather than from where you have been or where you are trying to get to.

*   *   *

You can't have a sense of being or doing outside of relationship.

On Being in Relationship

Go back to the basic truth: there is no way you can live outside of relationship. Period! In any good relationship, you willingly acknowledge the integrity of the person in front of you while maintaining your own integrity. Imagine a world where, every time you met someone, you would acknowledge this relationship.

* * *

Your student enters your teaching space, a person asking for help. They have needs, perhaps they have physical or emotional pain that they want you to address. They've asked many other people for help, and are hoping that you will have something different to offer, beyond what has been offered before. Without necessarily being aware of it, they seek information that will help them in their journey towards the fulfillment that will come in the absence of behavioral patterns that bind them to having to repeatedly experience their difficulties. Otherwise they would not have come to you — if the information they had previously received completely addressed their needs, they wouldn't need to seek further. What you have to offer that is distinct from most advice and practice is what you know about "use." For me, "use" or "appropriate use" means that you are behaving in accord with the way you are designed to function physically as your body reflects the quality of your thoughts, feelings, and perceptions given what you are doing. Or you are using yourself in discord with that design, given your commitment to patterns of behavior you might think you need to conform to who you believe you must be to be you. It's hard to choose the most appropriate response if you are riddled with habit. However, if I keep fostering the me I want to foster, I'll move closer to the me I really am. Or at least can be.

All the teachings from centuries past and current that we know — just to think of a few: Buddhism, Hinduism, Christianity, Islam, Judaism, and specific teachers such as Mother Teresa, Thich Nhat Hanh, the Dalai Lama, Marianne Williamson — they all give you tools for developing awareness about your position relative to yourself and what you are doing. You are then better able to decide whether the response you are swayed towards is the most appropriate one, given the evolution of your soul. Alexander's teaching does precisely that while offering a practical tool. You are trained in kinesthetic perception, i.e. how you organize kinesthetic impressions so you can recognize when your patterns of habitual behavior are compromising such an easy evolution of your soul. I'm not suggesting F. M. Alexander would necessarily agree with me on this last point, however many people might — especially in our century.

* * *

What might it look like to bring the Alexander work into simple acts of daily life? Perhaps you discover a moment where you become aware not just of what you're doing but how you use yourself to do it. What then? Do you set about correcting yourself, believing that giving directions will set all right? Instead of doing that, wait. Take a moment. All you are dealing with is time. And in truth, you have lots more time than you think. Time has lots of space. Then rather than trying to change, to become other than who you are most likely to be, enter the flow inherent in time and just allow yourself to meet yourself being yourself. You might be meeting yourself being yourself washing the dishes or having a difficult conversation with your daughter, your son, your spouse, your lover, your friend. Whatever or whoever it is, you are presented with an opportunity for you to see you for a brief moment. Perhaps you find yourself going down the road you've always taken and you know you need to choose otherwise but somehow you're going around the same old path once again. Just withhold defining anything — and decide if this is the self you wish to reinforce. Just take that moment of awareness and acknowledge being you in relationship. Simply say, "This is me having the experience of washing dishes, speaking with my daughter, or going down the habitual path once again." Because that is all that's happening on some very basic level. It means very little more than that. This is you having an experience. Forget defining your experience. Your experience of you having the experience will inform you better than you informing yourself using yourself in the same way that caused you to have to question the experience in the first place. This way leads to a better integration within you. It is reaffirming what already exists, i.e. you on a level beneath definition. Take that moment to locate yourself in space and time in relationship to whatever is going on.

*   *   *

The truth uncovered in a given lesson lies in the relationship between the teacher and the student. Insight is what happens, what shows up between you. It isn't the teacher imparting a truth to the student, saying, "If you live your life in accord with my teaching you will have all your questions answered." Rather, the truth of the lesson is what shows up in the process of meeting yourself being yourself without any expectation of what ought to be. This applies to the teacher and the student, both separately and together. At this point the teacher is more student than teacher, the student more teacher than student.

The more in contact you are with the quiet presence of your being, when receiving the student with your hands, the more you exist in relationship to something greater than and apart from your desires. You convey the same to the student, a sense of being at ease with themself, a more encompassing belonging. And when in this state, your touch remains unconditional.

When you have a conversation with someone, whether that conversation is verbal or kinesthetic, you have to really listen to the person speak. If you listen to them and know you have tapped into something deep, sacred, universal, the foundation of all life… when you have a conversation with someone who is really reaching out… there is a sacred trust. If you feel you are connected at that sacred level, you will be able to deeply communicate whether you know how to or not. Just listen. There is no greater gift you can give than to listen to another. Everyone wants to be heard, and should be, no matter what it is they need to say. And this is the person you touch.

I don't know what truth is, if there is a single truth. But the more deeply you embody the principles of being and of acknowledging relationship, then when you encounter another person, all you have to do is live there with them. They will show up proportional to their readiness and interest. You don't have to know anything about them, all you have to do is stay clear about your own commitment.

If there is one truth, it is that we exist in relationship. I always want to lead my life looking for the beauty of the person in front of me, sharing this relationship with me.

*　*　*

What we are teaching is a way of *being* in support while you *do*. Being while you do.

I do have an identity. But from time to time that identity gives way to the still point of support where I am just aware of being.

Any aspect of use of self — your experience of thinking and feeling and all that stuff — is reflected in the body. You cannot have an experience out of the body. Unless you leave your body but that is another discussion.

I started calling the work "Applied Practical Consciousness."

* * *

You start out as part of the ocean. You develop a set of behaviors that distinguish you from the whole — you become a wave. But you aren't separate from the whole. What if the wave decided that it wanted to exist forever in its current form and go off to have a cup of coffee! You develop a whole identity around that. But it can't be — the wave has to remain part of the ocean.

On Withholding Definition

We are often very quick to define a situation, person, or thing: "This is the delicious chocolate cake," "This is the boring staff meeting." But once we have defined whatever it is, we impose a filter between ourselves and it, a filter that preferentially lets in information that confirms our definition. In some sense, we are managing our experience based on our expectation, rather than letting the experience inform us. However, if we are able to withhold definition, even a little, we can allow in more information about the situation, person, or thing. Instead of wolfing down a second piece of chocolate cake because we have defined it as "delicious", we can actually taste it. Maybe it is too sweet, and we don't in fact like it. Or maybe it is indeed delicious, but having truly tasted it, we are satisfied with one piece. In listening to the colleague we have come to define as inarticulate and annoying, instead of tuning out or finding reasons to dismiss everything he says, we may find that today he has something important to say.

Withholding definition also applies in the realm of movement and physical activity. How often, at the gym, have you seen someone straining and bracing — almost before they have started to lift the weight? If we withhold definition regarding movement, we don't pre-determine the amount of effort that will be required. We don't pre-determine how we will do the movement — which muscles to use in which order. Instead, we set the intention for the movement or action as clearly as possible, and then let our system determine, moment to moment, what is actually required.

How does the concept of "withholding definition" differ from F. M. Alexander's concept of "inhibition?" In some sense, they are both very similar. They both, at root, have to do with refraining from reinforcing our habitual response to a stimulus. However, there are also a few differences. In his writings, and the writings of his students, F. M. appears to view inhibition as a kind of binary endeavor: you are either inhibiting, or not. Very often, as he and his students describe it, his students failed at inhibiting, causing a certain amount of frustration on the part of both teacher and student. In contrast, withholding definition is more flexible and fluid. You can think of it as lessening your commitment to your definition — you can always hold your commitment to a greater or lesser extent.

A second area of difference between inhibition and withholding definition is an area we might call "what next." Depending on which of Alexander's writings you are reading, once you are inhibiting you allow the teacher's hands to give you the right pattern; you give directions; or the right thing does itself. Whichever the method, the underlying idea seems to be that there is a right way to use yourself, and you are using different techniques to find it. When we come to withholding definition, in contrast, there isn't one correct way. Rather, we are always striving to interact, whether with the environment or other people, in a more fitting way. We want to continually fine-tune our responses and interactions in all our relationships. Withholding definition isn't a technique, but a mindset.

The next difference is a little slippery and subtle. It is one of emphasis, rather than content. In his writings on inhibition, Alexander most often focuses on inhibiting pull-down, or some sort of neuromuscular pattern. Of course, because of psycho-physical unity, the neuromuscular pattern belongs to an integrated whole that also comprises patterns of thoughts and emotions. However, for Alexander, the physical aspect seems to be the most common approach as a way in. Withholding definition, while also applying to the integrated whole, generally shifts the emphasis a little to the thought process as a way in. Just to be clear, both inhibition and withholding definition work with and affect the whole self. However, the conscious, cognitive part of the self can focus more on one aspect or another, as a way to broaden our understanding and appreciation of what we are up to.

Withholding definition, to whatever extent we are able to bring it into our lives, has tremendous power. If you have been up against a brick wall, withholding definition can allow a door to appear. Or at least a window.

*   *   *

I remember fairly early in my teaching career, maybe 30 years ago, a man came to see me because he wanted to break his habit of eating chocolate cookies. Around the same time, a woman came to see me because she wanted to drink only one glass of wine a night instead of three or four. This was before I had developed my ideas about withholding definition. I worked with each student with the more classical Alexander concept of inhibition.

Each person found that the addiction to the chocolate or alcohol kept them from actually tasting the wine or cookie. Immediate gratification, fulfilling the known was sufficient to fit the bill. Inhibiting let them actually taste the wine or cookies, and then they found that they didn't need to keep eating or drinking. That's how I did things 30 years ago.

A number of years later, long after the man had finished studying with me, he came back to see me because he wanted to tell me the rest of the story. It turned out that the cookie addiction was masking a deeper, much more serious addiction — one that nearly destroyed his life and relationship with his family. Looking back, I wonder — if we had worked with withholding definition instead of inhibition, would it have made a difference? Would he have been able to come to the point of saying, "Who am I?" and seeing the possibility of shifting his personal narrative? There's no way to know, but I wonder.

* * *

If you try to use yourself to solve a problem in the same way that you used yourself to create the problem, you will probably be left with the problem.

*   *   *

Withholding definition is about a certain fluidity of mind.

*   *   *

Withholding definition is an exceptionally nonjudgmental approach to teaching.

*   *   *

If I have recognized that I am habitually inclined to behave in a particular way, and I start to behave in that way, from a neurological point of view, I might need to inhibit in order to not do what I would habitually do. Alexander's process was to inhibit, and continue to inhibit while giving the directions. Direction was part and parcel of the inhibitive moment. Alexander would inhibit until he was satisfied with the results. I was not results oriented. What I'm exploring is the mystery of who I am. I'm not trying to solve the mystery. You can appreciate the mystery without solving it. That's how the idea of withholding definition developed for me. I objected to the results orientation too often sought in Alexander's inhibition.

*   *   *

If you inhibit — that is, you don't do what you usually do — you make yourself available to take in more information from what is around you. And what is a free neck if not freed from habitual neurological information? The moment you do not act as you are accustomed to doing, you allow the nervous system time to reset homeostatically. For F. M. Alexander, what you do when you inhibit is give directions. Withholding definition preempts and actually precedes and incorporates F. M.'s concept of inhibition. It allows you the time to consider more than usual, and while you give such consideration, your nervous system is strengthening your resolve.

* * *

The key part of the inhibitive moment for me is always that the person is in charge of the final outcome of the inhibitive act. For me, the inhibitive act is more a state of mind than something that you do. It happens the moment you become aware of what you no longer want to continue to reinforce.

* * *

Sometimes you must be lightning fast in defining — you must quickly step out of the way of the car bearing down on you. However, as you practice withholding definition, you will find that you are better able to define more accurately and see a larger picture because you have allowed more information to come in. Less is blocked from view in the absence of the anticipated. This information belongs both to your past experiences and to the conditions you are experiencing in the ongoing present. When you practice withholding definition, your definition of things will have a more encompassing reach in the present moment.

* * *

When you are willing to hold less need for definition, you are not attached to what you anticipate.

When you hold strongly to the need for definition, you are more attached to anticipating the outcome. Then it is less likely that you will see things from new insight, and moreover perhaps as things are.

On the Self

There are at least two aspects of self: the self in relation to what is going on, and the self as a constant.

Many people are always holding on to creating the self they think they need to be. We need to focus more on the self in relation to the environment in this moment. For you are only who you are at any given moment. This moment is the sum total of your identity. This fact was made clear to me when my wife died. On the last day of my wife's life, confined to bed, and unable to move without assistance, she suddenly asserted "I must stand up." She had been a dancer for all her life, and she wanted to experience standing alone without assistance for the last time, remembering how she had once done so easily, her feet tethered to the earth she so loved. The hospice attendant started to help her out of bed, but without success. I asked the attendant to let me assist my wife. I knew she wanted to experience standing from her own ability rather than being held up. So I reached across the hospice bed, and helped her rise in the way I might take a student off the table. In that moment, in a consuming and somewhat overwhelming epiphany, I understood that everything I had ever done and learned and become prior to this moment had prepared me to give my wife this one last gift. At that moment I existed for no reason other than to guide her towards her wish.

All I had ever experienced before prepared me for this moment — no other moment, simply this one, the only truth that could have possibly existed. I supported her desire to do the improbable, to stand on her own two legs that had only known dance for one last time. Then she fell back into her bed. I've never had that kind of experience, knowing that only in the moment where I was truly called upon to be me, that this was the sum total of my identity, where all who I had become had prepared me for the singularity of commitment to that moment. I felt truly blessed.

And, today because of this gift she gave to me, I remain blessed. Your job is to guide a person into the recognition of that moment when they understand that how they respond to any event in their life is who they are. Their identity is fluid and not fixed.

* * *

The "use of the self" is often seen in the context of what is universal, what is common to everyone. But it is also possible to look at the use of the self from the perspective of what is unique to each person. The uniqueness of each individual doesn't separate us, it unites us.

People often don't behave the way we think they should. We often don't behave the way other people think we should. If you really do uncover the use of the self, without any judgment whatsoever, it will be so much easier for you to move beyond where you don't want to stay. When I work with a person, all I try to do is give them who they can recognize at that given moment. You can observe and touch their uniqueness. You must, because each person is unique. Each person sees things in a way that is completely different from everyone else on the planet.

If you actually see the person as they are, they will change for they have been seen. People don't usually come to you because they want to find their uniqueness, but because they are in pain. The way you see yourself in the world is reflected in your use. When we give ourselves over to that which we think we need to do, generally we lose our sense of support. You want to get to the point where you can identify what it is about how you see yourself in the world that might be causing problems. The first step is just recognition, with no attempt whatsoever to do something about it. Change begins with awareness. Then inhibition — stop reinforcing the pattern.

The body knows where it needs to be to support what we want to be doing. The problem is that we put it where we think it needs to be — that is identity. However, it may not be the you you want to wave goodbye to the world with.

Once you define what the use of the self means to you, you go in one of two directions: either you get better at what you already are, what you are already doing, and improve your performance or, you discover new aspects of yourself that give you peace of mind. They're both valuable.

* * *

Identity, for me, is what the work is about — forging a deeper sense of who you are. You can be undefined but not without identity. In other words, you don't lose your Self when you release your need to hold onto your definition. You can withhold definition and still maintain your identity.

Most people want definition. Strong definitions creates rigidity. You can be rigidly moral, and you can be rigidly immoral.

* * *

Most people seem to have a secret longing to be more available to themselves. To be available to a deeper potential within yourself in difficult times is often superior to relying on what might have worked for you in the past -- what worked in the past might not befit present circumstances. To have this availability is equally attractive to those around you because you are modeling the advantages of reaching beyond your habitual response in favor of exploring potential, and finding a response that better suits the circumstances.

* * *

The first gift you are given is the gift of life. The second gift is the gift of self, the true, integrative self, that doesn't distinguish self from non-self, being a part of all that is. Nobody thinks, feels, or perceives exactly like you. If you steward this uniqueness, you will really explore who you are. The Use of the Self is a way of reclaiming the gift of self, which is the self you want to steward, the aspect of the self that is closest to you.

It is through the body that you experience the self while you are in the world.

On Compassionate Teaching

In France, they asked me, "How would you use your skills to work with Quasimodo[2]? He has a physical deformity that cannot be changed." I said, "When you look at Quasimodo, are you seeing poor use or a man in love?" If you put your hands on the person, on the man in love, you'll see where that could lead. If you put your hands on his deformity, his habit of identity, you will bind him to his pain of unrequited love given his physical limitations. No physical limitations limit your expression of self, of who you are. Quasimodo might very well have experienced a space within his physical limitations which allowed his capacity to love to extend far beyond how he previously had viewed himself.

* * *

You need empathy in order to understand compassionate response, but empathy alone offers little more than condolence. Compassion necessarily begins with empathy but within an understanding that commiseration offers no way out. Feeling their pain does little to resolve their pain. Compassion moves beyond empathy in offering something other than the expected. How do you let

---

2 Quasimodo, the hunchbacked character at the heart of Victor Hugo's novel *The Hunchback of Notre Dame*, is feared as a monster by the citizens of Paris, though he is actually good-hearted. His unrequited love for the beautiful Esmeralda is a central theme of the book.

go of a pattern of behavior? With compassion. Always with compassion. Embrace who you were when that pattern began, invite that person in, don't try to divorce yourself from the person you were. That is compassionate teaching as I see it. You would never see the possibility of who you might be without accepting all of who you have been. Such was your preparation.

It starts with self compassion. You can't really have compassion for someone else unless you have compassion for yourself. Remember when you first began training to teach it is you that you focus on and not the other. Don't lose yourself in the other; find yourself in the other for there you are — always.

On Bringing the Work to the Person

Much of the Alexander work is about giving the student an Alexander experience, usually with a dramatically changed sense of lightness in being and deep integration. Then this becomes their model to emulate. This is bringing the person to the Technique. But I believe it is at least, and perhaps more, relevant to bring the work to the person. You let the person show up, as they are — as prepared to resort to habit and as equally available to respond to a given stimulus in a completely different way. You let them choose while providing support for the availability to change.

The notion of letting the person show up will guide you into what to do next. Let yourself be surprised. The mysterious keeps showing up.

The moment I invite the diffusion of the localization of muscle tension using just enough pressure to stimulate the tissue to lengthen, I immediately look for how the student is processing the information. The moment belongs to the student. Once I start listening to the person, I belong to the experience.

On Finding the Fit

The idea for the term "finding the fit" came from a workshop I gave in Frankfurt, Germany. A participant in the workshop asked me for the key to unlock all the mysteries of the Alexander work. My response was, "I don't have a key, but if you start looking for locks, the key will show up." This led me to start thinking about touch fitting the person, in the same way that a key fits into a lock and the lock receives the key.

If you are looking for the fit, the first thing you think of is conforming your hand to the other's body part. But, you can also look for the fit without molding the hand: this turns into touch and be touched. What is touch and be touched? It is the acknowledgment that when we put a hand on someone to touch them, we are also being touched by them. You can only give what you receive.

Working with the fit leads to less doing. When you touch a person looking to find the fit, it involves a profound recognition of the integration of all life and the planet, similar to Thich Nhat Hanh's concept of *Interbeing* where each of us interacts with all life so that there is less to be done because all is in process of being done.

When you find the fit, you are finding the inter-relatedness of all patterns of movement throughout the body. If you conform your fit to keep fitting as the changes happen, the body will find its own still point of support given what it is being recruited for. If you keep conforming to the fit as the changes happen, *with the knowledge* that you want to keep free the head and neck to integrate everything through spinal flow, then you will get a deep integration. The deeper the integration, the more likely the student is to see who they actually are, and who they are creating because part of the nature of your design is to process the experience of what it means to be alive on the planet.

If you have trouble finding the fit, come back to yourself. How can you withhold definition more, really hear the other person. The more still you get within yourself, the better you will fit. Fit is the ability to let go of preconception and expectation in favor of what is most present.

Finding the fit is a means-whereby to meet the person where she is.

On Habit

_____

All habits are habits of identity.

*   *   *

How can we start to break free from habitual response?
The first step is simply to observe. To be witness to your
own interactions. Are your interactions always pretty
much the same? If you are always living in your habit,
it is very difficult to feel or experience your habit. When
you release out of it, then you can feel it.

To change your habit, you have to change your pattern
of use.

If your thinking really changes on a deep level, that will
change everything. The new thinking won't call forth the
old neurological and neuromuscular pattern.

On the Personal Narrative

We need to consider our personal narrative. We each have a personal narrative, and it is completely enmeshed in who we are and how we live. When we wake up in the morning, we wake up with our personal narrative, we don't wake up with our use alone. If I do yoga, I'm still doing it in a way that conforms to my personal narrative. It is the attachment to personal narrative that we are really changing when we change our use. Otherwise, we're just getting better at being the person we've been. And there is certainly value in this. However, if we really want to explore the mystery of ourselves, and encounter who we might actually be capable of being, we need to shift the personal narrative.

When I wake up in the morning, if I'm not really appreciative of my existence, I just get up and start my usual routine — coffee, shower, breakfast, work. The narrative is always there, seeping into everything we do. But for a moment in time, before jumping into that narrative, we can be aware of being. Very quickly, that turns into being aware of being you in relation to the environment and your narrative. When you first wake up, we almost immediately go to the narrative. But we do have a moment before commitment to personal narrative, and in this moment when your eyes first open and you acknowledge consciousness of your life in being alive one more day, you are closer to being than doing.

Try this exercise: When you wake up in the morning and begin another day on this earth, before you commit to personal involvement in another day, there might be a momentary awareness of being out of time before you commit to time. In this momentary preamble before there is a commitment to the activities of your day which give you reaffirmation of your identity, there might be only an appreciation of the mystery of you. And you simply momentarily lie where you have slept in this space between being and doing. There is no conflict, no uncertainty. In choosing the former you inhibit the latter. Not necessarily the other way around.

*   *   *

At the moment of conception the egg receives only one sperm, and that one is one among many. The egg and the sperm fuse into a single cell that quickly becomes 2 and 4 and 8, etc. You begin life on the planet! I think of this nascent beginning as the final outcome and the present stage of our evolutionary narrative, the story of our evolution as a species, and about the way in which we are designed to function while we process our experience of what it means to be a homo sapiens, a human being.

Our journey begins…

Our identity awaits us…

Our story begins…

Our identity becomes entwined with our personal narrative, which is both restricted and supported by our evolutionary narrative. The way in which we are designed to function, to process our experience of being human, began millions of years ago.

Our function is affected by our use. Our use evolves in context with social, economic, cultural, and genetic predispositions. Use also reflects both our attachment to our personal narrative, the story we tell ourselves we belong to, and the universal or evolutionary narrative. The personal and evolutionary narratives coexist. Because of this, you can reflect about who you might be, or wish to be, or have always been in your many incarnations, rather than be forever attached to a story that might not be reflecting who you really are. And this is where Alexander's discoveries pave the way for the freedom to change.

On Teaching from the Heart

Teaching from the heart is a state of mind. You use your hands differently. When the person comes in, most people don't have a real positive sense about themselves. There is a lot of blame, self-judgment. Even vanity is a type of disguise. "This is right." "This is wrong." "I'm not good enough." All these things. At the same time, Alexander asked the person to let go of a pattern of use which is reflecting their behavior, which they associate with being themself. "This is me, I can't change." And to change, you really need to truly see yourself. *Really* see yourself. Without an allegiance to the personal narrative associated with your identity. And so what I found when I was teaching in Europe for the first time was that people were willing to go further and deeper into simply seeing themselves with a great sense of clarity because they could feel that there was absolutely no judgment at all. No "this is right" and "this is wrong."

My wife once said to me when we were holding hands for no particular reason, except to share time and space together, "When you hold my hand I know all is forgiven." Now that's a beautiful statement. Not that there was anything to be forgiven, she simply felt seen and completely supported in that moment in her existence. I'm not suggesting that you, the teacher, hold hands with your students. However, your touch, the physical contact and exchange with your hands does certainly want to convey that no matter how inappropriate their use, in a sense "all is forgiven" and your time together is neither the beginning nor the end of their self-realization. In the training course, we did an exercise in which one student would work with another. Then they would stop working and just hold the person's hand while the person was thinking about something that was part of their life at the moment. The person in the teacher role was just there as support. There are receptors in the hand for love, for peace, for compassion, for social engagement. And then I would have the teacher work with the person from an Alexander point of view, having had the experience of their hands simply providing support, as we are designed to do. The difference for both teacher and student was palpable.

Teaching from the heart helps the person find total acceptance of whatever they have done. It helps the student to be able to look at choices, even bad ones, and the consequences of those choices, without a sense of identity. There can be so much shame.

On Support

_____

We are all designed such that our organism will support us given whatever we want to do. But, habitual patterns can interfere, making the body work harder than it needs to in order to keep us in support. We use an unreasonable amount of effort because we lose a sense of being in support.

*   *   *

Say you wake up in the morning, jump out of bed, and start your routine. You are doing things all day long. And then you end your day by getting ready for bed, and then you go to sleep. But for the most part, your life is a commitment to doing things as opposed to honoring a sense of being, apart from your desires. You do things based on desires. Life is fulfilling one or another small or large desire, over the course of a day, or a lifetime. In the absence of desire, you experience being in relationship to something apart from or greater than any desire you may have. And then you sense more of an inter-relatedness. The support comes from the inter-relatedness between yourself and all that is.

Recently I've been talking about the evolutionary narrative and your personal narrative. The personal narrative is pretty much determined by your sense of identity. And the evolutionary narrative is the story of evolution. Everything was designed to exist relative to another.

The evolutionary aspect of the narrative is that you belong to all of creation. You are part of creation. All life forms are part of creation. And it has little to do with your personal narrative. It is a narrative, there is a story to creation. We did not have identity for a long time — that came much later. The first part of creation is without identity. There is a book by Julian Jaynes, *The Origin of Consciousness in the Breakdown of the Bicameral Mind*. His idea is that there is no sense of personal identity in the *Iliad*. By the *Odyssey*, the idea has arisen that "I am responsible for my actions." At what point does the "I" come in — personal responsibility? Earlier, the gods are responsible for everything.

We, as the human race, favor doing over being. The Buddha tried to pull us away from that a little. That gives us a wider perspective. From the Alexander point of view, I distinguish between being and doing because in over-focusing on doing we tend to be taken out of support. We are designed to be in support while we are doing what we are doing.

On Observation

——————————

When you observe someone, you can look at them and/or see them. If you are looking at someone, it is possible to do so in a way that is projecting yourself. Alternatively, you can let the person show up. If you really take the person in, really see them as they are in that moment, they feel seen more closely for who they are in that moment and are more likely to see you.

One way of seeing a person is to see the parts: "Oh, look, I have changed the tensional dynamic of the musculature in your neck." But it isn't about parts, it is always about the whole person and how the way they use themselves physically reflects the quality of their thought, feeling, and perception. You want to develop ways of being able to see the whole of the person, how each part conforms to the whole.

Sometimes someone comes in and their parts aren't fitting well with the whole, but the potential is always there.

When you look at someone, you can see that which is restricted. If I have in mind: "She's using herself in the way I expect" — at some level, you are reinforcing your expectation. If you note the restrictions but see beyond them to the potential, that is different.

You need to meet the person knowing you don't know them.

Mother Teresa, Eckhart Tolle, and many other gifted teachers are "pulled down" in the Alexander jargon's sense of inefficient use of self. It's through the body that we experience self, while we are on the planet. Some people's minds are so strong and well developed that the body may not matter as much. Witness the life of Stephen Hawking. That's a fairly rare group of people.

When you are observing someone and their habit, you are really seeing their commitment to their habit. There is a difference between looking and seeing. Looking involves a lot of memory; you look through the eyes of what you remember and have defined. There is a real beauty in seeing and allowing yourself to be seen. Receive the other through your eyes that are present, through your heart that is present, and through your touch that is present, and let yourself be received. When you want to work with the potential of a person, you have to look at the person in a new way: you have to really see them.

When you observe someone, you may well observe misuse, that is, using yourself out of accord with how you are designed. However, you want to work with the potential, not with the misuse. You are not judging, but being reminded of what is possible.

Everything you observe is important. But if you only stay on the level of anatomy and alignment, you miss the other aspects of the person. If you limit your observation to what interferes with "good use," it won't be as useful to the person, because they will be less likely to fit their new experience into their narrative.

* * *

When you observe, you are stepping into an already moving river. There is nothing you need to do, or to make happen. When you step into the river, you accentuate the person's experience of being themselves.

* * *

Recently, I've been talking about the following: when a person walks in for a lesson, they should be seen for who they are, not looked at. Once you've made sure that you are safe in each other's company, before you look for the person's use, you are looking at their facial expression… look at the person well before you look at their use. There is already plenty written about mirror neurons and their functional role in determining immediate awareness of being safe in the company of someone you encounter. When you first see someone, there is a subtle definition that we make almost immediately. You watch someone tell their story. The pattern of use comes forth as they tell their story. If you put your hands only on their use, there's a subtle sense of judging the rightness/wrongness of it. But if they've been acknowledged as to how they feel, given their description of whatever has led them to see you, before you put your hands on them, there's a trust. The very first thing you want is for them to trust what you have to say, and you want to trust what you have to say. Their particular use belongs to them.

In the training recently, we've been watching a student play the violin. The trainees have been talking more about the state of mind of the musician, the feeling the musician has that is generated by the quality of their attention, rather than about the musician's use. The observation is not clinical at all. It's just that when you are really observing someone, you are looking at them with a knowledge that they don't have at that moment. You don't share that knowledge right away, until you have acknowledged them. We've been doing an exercise in the training in which everyone looks at each other. We notice that we have quickly defined the person we see in that moment. And the person feels defined, not seen. Then I ask them to look at the person again, and withhold definition, and see how much more information shows up about the person. Invariably, the person who is being observed does feel more seen than defined. We explore putting hands on the person having defined them, and then having gone through the other part of the exercise. Observation comes right out of withholding definition.

We carry around our own individual sense of identity. The other day I was listening to the news on the radio, and I heard a story about the Native American heritage of a politician. The news story was exploring the idea that our sense of identity is a social construct, and not science. An identity is social, not clinical — who you are relative to yourself, and to another. And how you are perceived by the other. The only thing that Creation did not give us is a way of seeing ourselves as others see us. So if you really want a good lesson, you try to squeeze your way into the middle of all that. Because it really is quite possible to see a person for who they are in a given moment.

Frank Jones[3] was really good at going right in there and making a change, and he brought the work to the person in a highly skilled way. And his words were filled with wisdom. One person's interference with that primary movement is not the next person's. They are all different. You encounter the difference given the degree to which they respond to what you give. Some people respond immediately, others are very slow in responding. And you touch things that you have no awareness that you are touching, that affect the person greatly. So observation has to be part of an ongoing continuum, because it changes during a lesson.

If you really see someone for who they actually might be, you have a much better chance of touching them in an appropriate way.

* * *

You don't want to look at someone in terms of parts, such as the head-neck-back relationship. I did an exercise in the training where you look at the predominant expression in someone's face — their base 'set', how their face is when they are not being affected by a particular

3 Frank Pierce Jones was a professor at Tufts University in Boston. He trained as an Alexander teacher with F. M. Alexander and his brother, A. R. Alexander. Jones carried out some of the earliest scientific studies of the Alexander Technique, which he described in his book *Body Awareness in Action*, Schocken Books, New York, 1979, reprinted in 1997 as *Freedom to Change*.

emotion. And then notice every other aspect of their body — their chest, ankle, jaw, every part of their body looks exactly like the predominant expression of their face. That observation clarifies that the person is whole and complete and when you see or touch one part of the body, you have touched the same thing in all parts of the body.

*   *   *

That which is observed does not go unaffected by the observer.

On Desire

_____

We are motivated by desire. Without it, we would be like the Buddha, with no problems. But in our lives on earth, we can't be completely without desire. The thing is not to be ruled by the desire.

If you take a moment to really experience the desire — for example, your desire to drink your tea — you will have a deeper experience than when only "satisfying" your desire.

*   *   *

When I talk about being motivated by desire, that is in the context of being and doing, and that is in the context of identity. The nature of our design is that you are designed to process the experience of being you, alive on the planet. Nobody makes the choices but you. When you use yourself more in accord with the way you are designed to process experiences, you make better choices: less judgmental and more inclusive. This gives you a deeper social engagement.

On the Role of the Teacher

When a person comes in, they come in with a need to be addressed. And you see them. If you are really hung up with use, then you will watch their use, look all over and see their use. There is nothing wrong with that, except that you are missing the boat. That's what F. M. Alexander was doing, and he had superior skills at changing and, to a large degree, correcting use. Even Patrick MacDonald[4] once told Alexander's biographer that Alexander was highly skilled at changing a person's use for the better, but that he had no idea who the person was he was touching, and this propensity exists today in the larger Alexander community.

It is different when you withhold definition. You meet a person with a need. That need is reflected in their use. Their use is reflecting their attachment to their personal narrative — that is the story you wake up with — the story of your life up till now — you know what you've lived. Most people are so attached to the story, that it is hard to step outside it. You can't live without a story — without it is a state like Alzheimer's — but you can be so committed to it that it is hard to see other perspectives

---

4 Patrick MacDonald was a graduate of F. M. Alexander's first teacher training program. He became one of the main first generation Alexander teachers, starting his own training course. MacDonald's training program influenced many other teachers who went on to lead their own training courses.

or access other potential possibilities. It's a habit of your identity. I cannot move the way you move, or think the way you think, nor do I have to.

So if you want to see the person who comes in, and have them be okay with having their pattern of use altered, you want to see the person reflected in their use, not necessarily or only their use reflecting the person.

There is flat out value in going up to someone and just working with their use. But if you stay in this profession for a while, you will likely get bored. The value of the work is sharing who you are. The value of any part of life is the same thing. The more you share, the more another shares. You are trying to be present for the person in front of you. The more present you are, the more present they are. I have always felt that a shared life is better than a life not shared. In giving what you know, you receive what you give from the other.

*   *   *

The teacher does what a parent does. The parent has lived through a lot of experiences. For example, crossing the street. You know how to do it, because you've done it. You don't say to the child, poised to cross the street by themselves for the first time, "Watch me, then cross the street." You take their hand and hold space for them to feel supported while they assimilate the necessary information to venture on their own. You "hold space," then, when you feel them process the information necessary, you let go.

An Alexander teacher needs to be sensitive to how much information the student can absorb and when they have absorbed it. When you ask them to let go, are you still there? If they don't feel you are there, they won't let go.

The teaching changes your way of being in dialogue with yourself. When I put my hands on you, it changes your relationship with yourself.

If this work is used to judge — if you are judging someone on the basis of what you think their use is — it cancels the entire value of the work. It is not about what their physical posture looks like.

Posture is a phase of movement. However, that phase can be extended and held consciously or unconsciously in matters of identity, i.e. who a person believes they need to be at a given moment. We can imagine a train of change going by, blowing its whistle as your signal to get on board. The train stops at every station but only for a moment. If one tightly holds onto a fixed way of being, thinking, feeling, or perceiving, as the train approaches one can refuse to get on board. One can watch the train go by, or one can get on the train. The train goes on without you. The ongoing present moves on without you. Remember a moment is a movement. And the "present" is but a moment you choose to belong to. You were given a ticket to ride at the moment of birth. You can remain "defined" as you wish to be and stand alone on the platform or step on board.

*   *   *

The martial artist trains by withholding definition over and over in order to know immediately when and how to move and for what benefit. You have to trust and believe in yourself that you will know what to do and when to let go. In the training, you take your time, withholding definition so that when the truly transformative moment comes you'll know exactly what to do immediately. Take joy in however you are able to show up in that moment, rather than being attached to the same story that repeats over and over.

Whatever you do as a teacher you can't use the work to challenge the person to give up what they know or think they know.

* * *

As you train to teach, you begin to clarify what the work means to you, and how to pass it along to another. Then you begin to clarify what the work means to you, really. You are, at the same time, inclined to pass it along to someone else, and also inclined to deepen your own understanding from a new perspective. If you don't give your gift — music, dance, etc. — it implodes. You have to give what you are.

> "You will understand what it means when you become what it means."
> Neale Donald Walsh, *Tomorrow's God: Our Greatest Spiritual Challenge*

In the end, all of the work is about you, and who you wish to share with another. You can run around looking for things — for love, esteem, etc. But really you just need to share who you are. You use all of what you learn in a training to discover and share who you actually are. Your security is your belief in yourself. You are the one who will be here until you croak, so be as close to your true self as you possibly can. Trust who you as a person have become through your willingness to grow and give away what you have learned. Trust yourself. For me the work, the teaching, is about learning to trust the ever-evolving birthing of yourself, and of appreciating the fluid nature of identity. Would you sleep through the night with someone you did not trust? I trust not.

*   *   *

In my life, my personal narrative was strongly shaped by birth trauma, but I didn't have an inkling of how this affected me until I had my first Alexander lesson with Frank Pierce Jones. At my birth, the attending doctor was drunk. The nurses pushed me back into my mother's uterus to delay my birth until the doctor was sobered up enough to deliver me. My first human contact was not welcoming. No loving hands gently cradling my headfirst introduction to the planet. My first human contact, the first touch I received at birth, conveyed rejection and betrayal: "go back, we don't want you." This rejection from the feminine energy (yin) of the nurses lasted a full hour and a half while the doctor was being sobered up. The next intrusion was a male energy, (yang) with a drunken high forceps delivery which left neurological scars. So on an energetic level I entered the world touched not with love and care but rather with rejection and betrayal and assault by drunken hands. For the first two days of my life it was unclear whether my mother and I would live or die. And so upon entrance I was a broken little boy and later an angry young man unconsciously holding the birth trauma of being rejected or betrayed by the feminine and hurt by the masculine. But this was not really me, and certainly not what I would have chosen to experience in life. To a tangible degree my birth experience affected the first 29 years of my life until I met Frank Pierce Jones. In my initial lesson with Frank my experience was that he was the first person ever to place hands on me from whom I felt no threat. However, until he touched me I had never known I had felt threatened. I was intrigued. The me who felt threatened was not the "entirely me" who walked out of Frank's office at Tufts University after that first lesson. Yet it took years to discover and process my reality. You teach who you are. You are guiding the person into a recognition that the way they are using themselves in the world might not be giving them what they really want. And you are guiding them into a deeply experienced recognition that the way they are behaving in the world is at least partly conditioned by their habitual ways of thinking, seeing, and feeling. All habit is habit of identity.

The Alexander work is about not completely giving yourself to whatever you define as your goal, the things you wish to accomplish. You don't need to go out there somewhere to find what really matters. The conundrum is that you think you need to be somewhere other than where you are. The answer is: you have to know that you already know. I don't give you anything that you don't already have. It's like giving directions: you don't ask your neck to be free because it's not free, you ask your neck to free because it already is free, although compromised. The absence of some degree of freedom would be your last breath.

*   *   *

Patrick MacDonald said that F. M. Alexander was really good at deficit-based pedagogy — he didn't use that phrase — that is, looking at what the student is doing wrong. That's how it was taught for so many years. It was highly critical and corrective. But that was the era. "I can get it in spite of them" — that was the thought. F. M. was very good at use — he knew exactly why he had his hands where he had them. But apparently he had no idea who he was working with. I received this same information from Frank Jones about F. M, and from Helen Jones, Frank's wife who also trained with both F. M. and his brother A. R.

Most people want to be seen and heard for who they really are, no matter how ineffective they might be in the moment.

With a deficit-based approach, we might be missing the person by focusing only on the use. We need to see the whole person. Look at the person's face, her expression. If you are able to look at your student, if you see their pattern of use, you'll see it reflected in their face. And you'll see vulnerability. And you'll see a person who doesn't need to be taught, but acknowledged and guided into being more close to who they actually are.

To really look, we need to withhold definition. We all totally want a definition. And there is nothing inherently wrong with that. Except that the definition is usually right next to you — but you want it so much that you aren't in the present. You are already anticipating not having it. But it is already with you. That is what you are teaching — as far as I'm concerned, that is the Alexander Technique.

*   *   *

What do I teach?

Practical consciousness — applied.

Alexander taught the Alexander Technique. Perhaps he was the last to do so.

I teach my vision of a better world. I think Alexander had the same notion in mind.

I have been greatly influenced by the lessons I learned from Frank Pierce Jones, among them his views about teaching Alexander's discoveries without necessarily following exactly in his footsteps. In his book *Body Awareness in Action* Jones wrote:

> The aim of teaching, as I conceive it, is to bring a pupil to the point of self-discovery that F. M. reached when he was able to translate what he saw in the mirrors into kinesthetic terms and to apply his new knowledge to the solution of his own problems and become in effect his own expert in the use of himself. To accomplish

this result I do not believe it is necessary, or desirable, or for that matter possible to follow the same steps that F. M. followed in making his discovery or that I followed when I began studying the technique. My aim is to give my pupil as quickly and surely as possible the benefit of my present knowledge and understanding and help him avoid the false starts and misconceptions that slowed my own progress.[5]

I question teaching the Alexander Technique as something to aspire to, using the "directions" to measure up to a standard of behavior you are not yet ready to embody. I teach consciousness and its practical application to life as a way of meeting yourself being yourself and deciding in any given circumstance if the "you" you customarily ascribe to being is the "you" you wish to be in the present circumstances. And I use Alexander's insights to demonstrate how to apply your consciousness to exploring the mystery of who you might be apart from who you think you need to be in any given moment. This would be the inhibitive moment — Eugen Herrigel's Zen archer's moment of highest tension, who when "standing before the target (a reflection of himself), very much aware of where the target is in relation to what he seeks to accomplish, draws back the bow and just at the moment he is most apt to hold on, he lets go."[6]

* * *

---

5 *Body Awareness in Action,* Schocken Books, New York, 1979, p. 153. The book was reprinted in 1997 under the title *Freedom to Change.*

6 *Zen in the Art of Archery*, Rutledge and Keegan Paul Ltd, London, 1953, p. 35

Be less of a teacher and more of a student. You are the teacher, but only proportional to the amount you are willing to learn.

It certainly helps when teaching to be a witness to your student experiencing what they are experiencing.

On What the Teacher is Teaching the Student

My current way of defining what I teach is, I believe, a way of paying homage to Mr. Alexander. In my teaching, I focus on the series of discoveries he made which at first were based on solving a problem that no one else could solve, i.e. his vocal problem. His method of addressing his long-standing vocal problem was successful, and so he turned his technique of addressing recovery into a teaching. I often suggest that only F. M. Alexander taught the "Alexander Technique." So my focus when teaching is on his series of discoveries which ultimately led to the technique. This is what I mean by homage. The teacher is basically introducing the concept of "use" to their pupil, which, if adequately understood, can literally transform their life. The teacher explains how by using their kinesthetic sense of perception, the student can be aware of not only what they are doing, but also of how they are using themselves to do it. The student is guided into a method for observing themselves, and seeing behavior patterns. If you use yourself too far out of accord with how we are designed to function, you will run into problems. The teacher guides the student into finding the patterns.

With hands-on work, the student experiences a general level of appropriate muscle tone in their body which gives them a feeling of lightness and integration. People tend to chase that feeling, always wanting to find it again. And pupils become used to what they expect from their teachers. You won't have that exact experience again. Your first experience is opening the door. After that, don't look for the experience you had, look for the experience you are having. What the Alexander work can be used for is to help you stay in the ongoing present: "How deeply committed can I be to the experience I am having?" In my work with another I am less interested in the habit except as a point of reference or a gateway to an underlying depth of support. It is this world beneath and with the "conditions present" that I seek to touch.

There is the familiar, the habitual, that the person comes to a lesson with. It is heavily biased toward doing. When you are more in the being mode, it is more about relationship with something apart from your desires, not necessarily exclusive from individual desire but certainly connected to a wider and more encompassing availability. Within the being is the person's potential, and you are touching them to remind them of that. We are all used to the known. But there is more to us than the known.

How would you work with someone so that they experience their potential, rather than the habitual? That is our raison d'être as teachers. In addition to communicating that through the hands, also explain it verbally, how it might be useful to them. When you talk and answer questions, stay with yourself as the teacher. Whether or not you have hands on, it is the same relationship. You are staying with yourself, and receiving. You can only give what you can receive.

On Stories

We all have a story. When you meet people for the first time, you swap stories. You tell those stories that have helped shape who you have become. Your story is based on your quality of experience. The nature of your experience affected you in such a way that you feel it shaped your life. You have a composite of stories. Usually there is a thread of consistency. However, if I use myself to tell my story in the same way that I went through the experience, I'm not using what I learned. If you spend your life doing that, you have an adaptive pattern of use that doesn't let you take in what you have learned.

I first started to do story work when working with actors when I was a faculty member for 12 years for the Institute for Advanced Theater Training, American Repertory Theater at Harvard University. At the start of each semester, I asked the actors in the class to tell me a little about themselves. I got all kinds of glowing, pie-in-the-sky narratives. I thought, they are all very much the same. They are all using themselves in a way that the gestures aren't really theirs. But I'm not here to tell them that. So I said, tell your story. Then I worked with them, and asked them to tell the story again. They all came out really differently. It changed their whole method of learning and not necessarily just in my classes but in the whole Institute. They were all a wonder to watch grow.

After that, I tried it in workshops, starting in Ireland.

Everybody has a story. You wake up to the story you have been living. You come out of the womb and nurse. You are your mother's breast at that moment, because you don't have a sense of the other. Most of your development comes from touch. That is primary. Touch is amazing. We are designed to touch everything. We are designed to touch each other. Not to manipulate through touch, but to inform and be informed.

There comes a time when you are not your mother's breast. You hear sounds, you see things around you. But you aren't what you see and hear. Then who are you? You spend the rest of your life engaged in that little exercise. "Who am I if not the other?" And then your story begins.

You are filled with stories all your life. Some of them are deliberately repressed. The body does that too — for example, repressing memory of pain of childbirth. There are stories that pop up when you aren't even aware of them. There are other stories you keep retelling and they form the fabric of your identity. We feel it is easier to be the one we feel we need to be. When we touch someone in an Alexander lesson, we can use our touch to let the person come closer to who they actually are, rather than the story they think they need to be.

The story we tell each other comes out of relationship, and that's important. We think it is our own story, but it is our story in relationship. Which means that change happens in relationship, it doesn't happen out of relationship. You can rewrite your story. It is difficult to rewrite the story without changing your use.

If you look at pictures of Alexander, it is difficult for me to believe that a lot of the time he wasn't aware that he was being photographed, and was as upright as possible. Changing your use doesn't mean that you have to always look like you are Alexandrified. It means that you are fluid — fluid of response, fluid of identity. We are mostly fluid. But we don't think of ourselves as fluid. But when you put your hands on someone you can feel the fluidity.

*   *   *

When you work with someone, can you distinguish between someone's personal narrative and their use? Are they so deeply into their personal narrative that they can't see other possibilities? Through their use you can touch their personal narrative. If you can do that, the work stays interesting because people are always showing up.

It's the attachment to the narrative that stifles the fluidity of your identity. And then something happens and it throws you off, and then it's like, wow, it's a whole new life. It's the attachment to the story that you want to be able to sense — when the person is attached to the narrative, and how it is affecting their use.

*   *   *

When you tell your story, you can either re-create the conditions that created the situation, or you can use what you have learned.

When a person comes to see you when they are in pain, they are looking for information that will help them. When they tell their story, they are usually using themself in the same way they did to create the pain. Then the teacher works with them. The idea is to tell the story from who you've become, rather than who you remember yourself to have been.

Taking responsibility is empowering. In every moment you have choices. It's not blaming everything on external forces.

The Alexander teacher provides that little bit of support to allow the person to do what they really want to do.

When someone is telling you an important story, you listen completely, but without getting lost in their pain. You are there to give support, not commiserate. Commiserating is getting lost in the fray. Compassion is offering another alternative.

Let's say you are grieving. If you are contracted into a pattern of use, you'll feel the grief, but you won't experience it deeply. So you end up having to experience it again. You have to open yourself to really experience the grief.

When you put your hands on someone, in a sense you are putting your hands on their story. The condition of the tissue reflects everything that has happened to them.

Your personal story is not complete without sharing it. A story can't be in isolation, it's part of the universe. You can tell if the story they are telling is the real story. If there is a feeling of agitation, it's not yet the deep story. When you are with the deep story, it gets real quiet.

* * *

As I mentioned, we all have stories. Some of those stories have helped shape who we have become. I'd like to share one of my stories, a formative story.

I grew up in the southern portion of the United States, where in 1960 schools, restaurants, movies, water fountains, etc. were still segregated. In other words the white and the black person were segregated from communion. If you were black you simply were not allowed to believe that you could eat next to someone in the restaurant if they were Caucasian, or drink from the same water fountain, sit together at the movies, or swim in the same swimming pool, etc.

This was a way of life that had existed for many, many years. Although some certainly always questioned this as a way of life, the majority of people simply grew up living this way. If you were white you seldom overtly questioned it. If you were black you were not supposed to question. However, in the sixties, in Bob Dylan's view, *the times they were a changin'*. And Martin Luther King was just around the corner.

I was eighteen years old. And I had an experience quite similar I think to an Alexander lesson where, as the events unfolded, my experience of being me was elevated beyond my comfort zone and into an experience of myself that canceled out all habituation of thought, feeling, and perception. And this brought me into an awareness of who I actually was or certainly might be and simply could not deny. You might say in our parlance that my neck was freed from the yoke of cultural bias which I was born into, that really had nothing to do with who I was.

The incident happened at a local drive-through hamburger stand one night when maybe 10 carloads full of high school students from my high school were gathered. In those days you would sit inside your parked car, seated in pairs or as many as a car would hold, or you would stand outside of your car talking to classmates. You drank Pepsi, Dr Pepper, or Coca-Cola and you ate hamburgers, french fries, and hotdogs.

Essentially you were having a good time. You were a teenager, and you were rowdy and you made a lot of noise. So the parking lot of the hamburger stand was filled with all of us having a good time making conversation. We were living our lives of expectation. We were clearly defined. We were comfortable in being ourselves. And, *the times they were a changin'.*

For two carloads full of black women and children drove into the parking lot. They parked their cars, got out of their cars, and slowly walked toward the serving window of the hamburger stand the purpose of which was to be served just like the rest of us. Once the women and children got out of their cars, immediately, the entire parking became quiet and very still. No one was making noise anymore, no one was talking. We were all busy observing what was taking place, which from our cultural upbringing was not supposed to be taking place.

Two carloads full of black women and children stood before the serving window. They were asking to be served. The manager of the hamburger stand, crossing his hands back and forth signaled, "I can't serve you." They must've asked again. For he signaled again, crossing his hands once more, and with some degree of frustration he mouthed, "I can't serve you." There was a pause, a very long pause before the women, thoroughly humiliated, turned to look at each other then slowly began to walk away one by one. The parking lot was completely quiet, no sound was made. Only observation. Individual and collective experience.

Then, one of the women, the one who placed the order, as she turned away she tripped and fell to the ground. The silence broke, and the parking lot, filled with teenagers, broke into laughter. The women and the children froze; no one moved.

Except for me. I moved, not really knowing why except that I too knew humiliation, I too knew what it felt like to be laughed at and ridiculed. Who, among all of us teenagers, gathered around our cars and now laughing, who among us had not known humiliation?

Within moments I stood next to the woman who had fallen. She wouldn't look up at me even when I extended my hand to her. And, once I extended my hand the entire parking lot became quiet again, immediately. All was silent again, still and silent.

She neither looked at me nor took my hand. I spoke to her, "Take my hand." I smiled. Still not looking at me she took my hand. I lifted her up, and standing facing each other we looked into each other's eyes briefly, and forever, each uncertain how to respond to our unexpected encounter and then I and the black women and children walked together toward their parked cars. Everyone got back into their cars, women and children, respectively. I opened the door for the woman with whom I walked. Neither of us had words for what we were experiencing. Before I assisted her into the car we looked at each other, both with an understanding of what had and was taking place and with disappointment in life as we had just experienced it. I think she thanked me. I think I nodded my head affirmatively but I had no words. I was overtaken by the sheer nature of an all-consuming and unanticipated experience. I closed her car door. They drove away, the two carloads full of women with their children. They simply drove away. I watched them drive away. And they were gone as quickly as they had driven into the parking lot.

And I became aware that I was standing alone, divided between the cars driving away and the cars parked and filled with my classmates. I stood alone with my back facing my high school classmates. At that moment,

I realized as I stood alone watching the women and children drive away, that I could never go back to what was behind me. The awareness was coupled with an insight that I had just left what had been a belief I had seldom questioned and had never encountered as I had just done. I had just left my past. I could not really turn around again and see things the same way as I saw them now. Any one of us could've extended our hand to that woman lying on the pavement. It was simply what you do. A person is humiliated, they fall down and lay further humiliated from their falling on the pavement and you simply extend your hand to help them up. It's that simple. So why didn't more than one person perform that action, why didn't more of us go to help her regain her dignity as a human being? What happened should not have happened. And yet it did.

As I stood alone looking at all my classmates, I was consumed with a new awareness of belonging and not belonging. Belonging to something apart from who I had thought myself to be, I stood undefined but not without identity. I came to a very deep understanding in that moment when looking towards my classmates, who still remained silent, even until I got into my father's car to drive home, that I could never be anyone except who I was, and that was yet undiscovered.

This is my experience and my response to it. It has become one of many stories that helped shaped who I have become well before I was ever exposed to the Alexander teaching. However the stages of awareness and learning born from the experience do resemble an

Alexander lesson as I have had them and as I have given them.

First, I was given an experience of being me apart from the way that I was accustomed to being me. Second, the experience gave me a new awareness of potential. Third, the experience joined with a new insight of who I might be rather than who I felt I needed to be to be me. Fourth, the experience gave me a deeper understanding of myself. These are the four stages of learning one can be guided through in any given lesson. And in fact on a good day they all happen together, "each one separately and all at once."

After the women and children drove away, I got in the car with my best friend at that time. And he said, "What the hell did you do that for?" I looked at him for a long time then replied, "How could you not do that?" He said nothing and I drove away. And based upon this experience, this lesson which wove together all of my misgivings about how I had grown up and how I might yet evolve, months later I left my home state, went to California and embarked upon a career in theater that was as far from my expectations as I might ever have considered. But that's another story.

On Using Your Hands

If you just listen to the body when using your hands, you won't have the person. But if you listen to their response to what you are conveying, you'll have more of them.

You can practice using your hands all day long, if you use your consciousness when you touch something. To practice the aesthetic of the hand, the hand belongs to the arm, the arm belongs to the torso, and altogether they belong to your mind.

*   *   *

When you place hands on a student, you are placing hands momentarily on habit. The person is accustomed to over-recruiting, holding themself up. But only for a moment do you linger with that initial feel. Instead, you listen beneath and within their habituation and you will discover a movement that belongs to the way in which the person has been designed to function. If you were to use an analogy of the wave and the ocean, you will note that the wave distinguishes itself from the ocean, rising up clearly as a wave. However the water in the wave always sinks back into the ocean before standing out again in the next wave. Not so with the habit, where an individual need to distinguish oneself apart from the whole and hold onto that identity tends not to return to the ocean [wholeness] as readily as nature's waves, absolved of any identity, might return.

When you make contact with someone, you are touching a moment. You are helping them identify what it is that they no longer wish to reinforce, and sense other possibilities.

* * *

Not everyone will feel the changes. There may be a legitimate reason for that — it's never the student's fault. You just have to find another way to reach them.

* * *

Ultimately, we want to work as close as possible to the intention. Closest to not doing. Working through your intention is a path to choosing not to do. If I, as a teacher, really let you show up in every way you can be, you do most of the work — which is the heart of it.

* * *

You can work with the specificity of the relationship of the head and neck to the whole, and that will affect the whole. As you work more comprehensively, it involves deeply acknowledging what *is* — no judgment, no desire to change, just acknowledgment.

Working with non-doing hands involves really trusting the design of us. The design of us is designed to keep us actively in relationship. If your goal is to communicate to the person their own deep, abiding integrity, rather than a bundle of habits, you recommit to your own integrity and believe and trust it — that is sufficient.

*   *   *

What I put my hands on is movement. I think of the presence of movement (freedom) and the absence of movement (restriction).

On Touch

Generally, in our culture, when a person touches another, they want something in some way. The touch is conditional. Most touch is one person attempting to get another person to agree with their reality, to agree with their vision of the world. There is some degree of manipulation involved, however minor.

The touch we want in Alexander is unconditional. We don't want anything. Instead, we want to touch someone while letting ourselves be touched. How deeply can you be touched by the inherent beauty of someone else's being.

When you touch someone in a non-doing way (that is, a non-manipulative way), it is two intelligent systems talking to each other. If you are integrative in your own use, you will communicate that to them. When I touch a student, I listen to the movement beneath the pattern of behavior, to the ocean beneath the wave. That is the more integrative movement.

Listening and receiving are states of being that you want to bring to your work. Part of the quality of the touch is the knowing — for example, deeply knowing about the head-neck relationship, knowing what is possible for humans as they move away from what they habitually do.

*   *   *

As we've seen, we each have our own stories, stories that combine to form the personal narrative that makes us who we are. The following story is a part of my personal narrative, one that informs my understanding of the power of touch.

Quite a few years ago, when teaching a workshop in Japan, I had a remarkable experience. I had been teaching in Tokyo and Osaka for two weeks. The next day I would return to Boston. There were fifteen participants in the workshop, none of whom had previously experienced an Alexander lesson, and none of whom spoke English. I decided to give each person a brief encounter with the work through demonstration with hands on. I came to the third person, a young woman of perhaps twenty-one years old. She was sitting in a typical zazen position on the studio floor, with folded legs and hands and a slightly slumped spine. I asked her permission to let me place my hands on her head and neck. I stood behind her while she remained sitting. My translator conveyed my instructions in Japanese. Her response was immediate. Her spine first lengthened and she settled, then she turned to look at me as if she were awakening to a new experience of herself.

I asked her about her experience. Only a few moments had passed since I first touched her.

"I don't feel as though I should be hit," she replied.

"What do you mean?" I asked, not really following her reply.

"Before you touched me, I have always felt I should be hit," she said.

I stepped back away from her and asked pretty much the same question I felt everyone else in the studio was asking themselves in that moment, "What do you mean?"

"My parents beat me."

"You mean when you were a little girl?"

"No, now," she replied.

I spoke from direct concern: "Are you aware that you are inviolate, that no one has the right to hurt you or harm you?"

"I know that now," she replied, "but I did not know this until you touched me."

We had known each other for a few minutes. We smiled at each other. "Can you make me a promise?" I asked.

"Yes," was her reply.

"When you feel safe enough and you are with your parents, I want you to stand before them and speak to them quietly and say in a simple way, 'I am inviolate. No one has the right to hurt me or harm me. And you've never had the right to hurt me or harm me. And if you ever harm me again, I will leave and you will never see me again.' Then ask, 'Will you harm me?'"

She was silent, calm. She simply smiled and looked at me. "Can you say this?" I asked.

Then, without a moment's hesitation, "I can now... now that you've touched me."

Touch... Unconditional touch on some deep level of communication frees one from all false sense of self belief. She was no longer the person who had been conditioned to believe she was a person who deserved to be hit.

I flew home the next day. And I returned to Japan the following year to teach again. And of course I wondered if I would I see this young woman again? She showed up for a private lesson with her translator, and carried with her a briefcase and two large poster boards. She was smiling. Speaking to me through her translator, and with authority, she said:

"Sit down."

Her smile grew as I dutifully obeyed and sat down.

Then she presented the first poster board. On the poster board she had transcribed in meticulous Japanese characters four generations of Japanese families with dates of marriages, parents, grandparents, great grandparents, children, and grandchildren replete with dates of marriages, births, deaths. She then explained the violence in all four generations.

"This was my family."

Then she directed my attention to the bottom of the poster board and pointed to where she had written her name.

"I don't belong to that family anymore. I live here," she said, pointing to her name written off the generational chart. "I kept my promise."

She explained that she had stood before her parents and repeated verbatim what I had suggested she say to them: "I am inviolate. No one has the right to hurt me or harm me and you've never had the right to harm me and if you harm me again I will leave and you will never see me again. Will you harm me? I told them this. And they replied they would not behave differently."

So she got a job, left home and found an apartment.

She presented the second poster board to me. On this poster board there were perhaps thirty small clouds drawn. Within each cloud was a text, the first of which read: "I am inviolate. No one has the right to hurt me or harm me."

On that first cloud, she had written what I had told her was her birthright. As another self-realization materialized, that went into the next cloud, and then another, and then another. With each successive saying she would meditate until she was secure in realizing who she actually was and not who she had been conditioned to believe she was.

"Now I only see my parents on special days, out of respect and only in a crowded restaurant. I am my own woman now." She smiled an exceptionally genuine smile and said: "And it is your fault!"

Then she placed the poster board down and exclaimed: "I would like a lesson now."

And I thought to myself, "Yes, I will gladly return a lesson in kind after the lesson you just gave me."

Touch!

Beneath and within any given person's being is a sacred space of safety, of self-love and worth, of who you actually are and have always been and not who you think you need to be to be you.

On Working in Activity

You end up working with the person's involvement in the activity, with their experience of being who they are while involved in the activity. While doing that, you need to also be committed to where you are relative to what you are doing. That's the Zen archer — poised between being and doing.

You never want to take the person away from their involvement in the activity. It's like entering a stream and going with the current, rather than staying stationary and having the current flow around you.

In placing hands on someone involved in an activity, you are inviting a choice in the movement — to do what you usually do, or something different. You can put your hands on her involvement with who she thinks she needs to be to sing the song. You aren't just working with the body, or with use, but with the *self*.

*   *   *

When you work with someone in activity, you want to help the person be more embodied while they are doing whatever they are doing. Emphasizing the habit, to call it out for inhibition, will tend to stop the person. Any whiff of criticism will be unhelpful. When I watch and listen to someone sing, I don't think about the Technique. I just appreciate, whether the person is accomplished at singing or not. The traditional Alexander approach is to help the person inhibit habitual use. I prefer to appreciate what the person is doing, and be moved to join in. You can't really separate the use from the person, but you can emphasize use at the expense of the person. It is critical not to judge yourself or the person — that clouds things. Meet yourself without judging.

*   *   *

It is not my right to remove you from where you are. It is my right to reveal to you where you are, without removing you. Once you know where you are, you will move wherever is available to you to go, if you want to.

On the Primary Control

F. M. Alexander wrote to Frank Pierce Jones that there really isn't such a thing as Primary Control: "There really isn't a primary control as such. It becomes a something in the sphere of relatively." Frank had written to Alexander in an attempt to be clear, when discussing the technique, about how he explained primary control. Frank's research focused on cervical and occipital reflexes that do indeed affect the total pattern of neuromuscular movement throughout the entire organism. However Frank was very much aware in his thinking at the time of his research that there are numerous other controlling mechanisms that are involved in the process described by Alexander as primary control. Personally, I prefer Frank's view of primary control as the head and neck reflexes facilitating the voluntary as opposed to the voluntary impeding the reflex.

* * *

The master key (the primary control) is relationship. To me, primary control is the awareness of relationship. Is there an actual primary control? I have no idea why Alexander used this phrase. I do know that he never used it until Rudolf Magnus conducted his experiments on tonic head-neck reflexes in animals and humans. Based on his experimental results, Magnus concluded that the head-neck reflexes are the consequence of a change in the position of the head in relation to the trunk, and have substantial bearing on righting reflexes which are situated in the brain stem. Alexander seems to have adopted Magnus's experiments as conclusive proof of controlling mechanisms belonging to the head's relation to the rest of the organism, and he decided to label this relationship "primary control."

Many teachers feel there is no primary control as such, but there is a specific relationship of head to neck to non-restrictive and healthy spinal functioning which affects the organism as a whole, and does indeed affect our movement in response to gravitational force. I do know there is a movement that is primary insofar as the head needs the freedom in the neck muscles (which really extend into the head and the back) to move at the atlanto-occipital joint. In a research paper, Blandand and Boushey[7] describe the cervical spine as being "the most complicated articular system in the body … normally the neck moves over 600 times an hour, whether the individual is awake or asleep" — that's an average of once every 6 seconds! "No other part of our musculoskeletal system is in such constant motion."

---

7 *The Cervical Spine, from Anatomy and Physiology to Clinical Care*, Blandand and Boushey (1992), one of 115 papers presented at the 1989 International Union of Physiological Sciences Conference in Fontainebleau, France and published as the book: *The Head-Neck Sensory Motor System* (Berthoz et al, 1992)

My old friend, David Gorman[8], put it very well in a recent letter to me:

> I think it is worth noting that it is not the so-called 'neck', as in "free your neck", which is the point here. The whole reason why the neck is what it is, and why it has such a flexible range of motion, is because of your head. You cannot move your neck by itself. Try keeping your head and shoulders still, and then somehow move your neck. You cannot do it. This is because your neck is not so much a thing in itself, rather, it is the junction between your head and the rest of you. Your neck is the limb for your head — it's your head's way of getting around.
>
> And why is it so essential that your head has that huge range and freedom of movement afforded by your neck?
>
> Your head isn't just that roundish bony thing with hair on top. It's where most of your outer-directed senses are located, especially the ones which detect what is going on at a distance, such as sight, hearing, and smell (as contrasted to touch which needs direct contact). Furthermore, these senses are not just passive receptors taking in what comes to them, like a camera or a microphone. Instead, you the person, are constantly and actively seeking out information — turning to look, following a lovely scent with your nose, cocking

---

8 David Gorman is an Alexander Technique teacher and trainer of teachers, as well as the founder of the LearningMethods work. He is also the author and illustrator of several books, a 650-page anatomy text, *The Body Moveable,* and a book on the Alexander Technique, *Looking At Ourselves*, as well as many other articles and essays.

your head to pinpoint a sound, or following someone's movement and then smiling and using your voice to respond to them. As you give attention to the world, your head is constantly moving, gathering information about what is happening so that you can respond. And as you respond, your head is moving to lead and guide your intended activity.

In other words, it is the job of the neck to provide the huge range of motion needed to follow your head — i.e. your attention and intention — so you don't have to turn your whole body every time you turn to look at something. As well as enabling your head movements, the neck's muscles also simultaneously support your head as it moves. Equally importantly, your neck muscles and joints are absolutely loaded with sensory mechanisms constantly reporting to your system where and how your head is moving so that the whole rest of you knows what you are getting into and therefore can be organized to follow your attention and intention into activity in a coordinated, supported, and balanced way.

Accordingly, the saying that your 'head' leads and your 'body' follows is not really accurate; it's your attention and intention which lead and the rest of you is then coordinated into your activity and into the world.[9]

∗   ∗   ∗

---

9 Private communication with David Gorman, 27 July 2019. Printed with permission.

When we work, we aren't working with the primary control so much as working with what is interfering with the body's predisposition to homeostasis.

*   *   *

The neck is the key and the lock is the self. You have to turn the key the right way to open it.

On Directions

The primary directions are: neck free, head forward and up, back to lengthen and widen. They are primary because they affect the whole organism.

*   *   *

Does giving or affirming a direction actually initiate the movement inherent to the direction? No. It is true that giving a direction is essentially setting an intention, and the nervous system does indeed organize the organism around a person's intentions. However, from the brain's perspective, giving the direction "forward and up" does not actually cause the head to move forward and up. Rather, the moment you give a direction to yourself, you are no longer doing what you were doing a nanosecond ago. And in the absence of whatever you were asking your nervous system to do, the nervous system leans towards a homeostatic response given what you are doing. For a brief moment you are not totally buying into your habit.

*   *   *

Directions are like vitamin pills. We can take them as a precaution.

*   *   *

It's far better to meet yourself being yourself in the moment, rather than trying to constantly live up to the directions.

The Buddha did it through inhibition, though he didn't call it that. The Bhagavad Gita is one huge book about an inhibitory process.

*   *   *

I've always been intrigued by the apparent difference between Hillel's (one of the most important Jewish religious leaders), and Jesus of Nazareth's (the central figure in Christianity), version of the same admonition. Hillel suggested that we do not do to another what we would not want done to us. Jesus suggested that we do unto others what we would have done to us. Both admonitions amount to the same thing. However, with Hillel we are asked to inhibit the former and thereby choose the latter. And with Jesus, we are asked to choose the former and thereby inhibit the latter. Two versions of inhibition.

It is interesting that in both formulations, the concept of inhibition lies in the thought process, exclusive of the body. F. M. Alexander went a step further and included the embodied self. What if we were to take it yet one step further and also include the concept of withholding definition? What if, for at least a brief moment, we withheld definition about how our actions would affect someone else, and also withheld definition about how we want them to treat us? That could allow time and space to let the other show up and to see them, while letting oneself show up and witnessing oneself. The resultant choice would come from a self-generated expanded awareness.

* * *

If direction works for you, use it. If it works in specific circumstances, use it there, in that moment. I believe Alexander meant to use directions together with inhibition, not separate from it. When Alexander first realized that he could not prevent himself from succumbing to his habitual way of speaking by *doing* things differently, he realized that he had to *let* his neck be free. A huge moment of awareness. He realized that he must allow the unfolding actions of the moment to take precedence over his accustomed way of thinking. That accustomed way of thinking was compromising the freedom needed in his neck muscles. For me, initially it was all about inhibition. The moment I was able to stop doing what I noticed I was doing, I immediately found a deeper movement. Later, I found withholding definition more all-inclusive as a means-whereby.

The body knows what it has to do. The body will find a way. You let it be your guide as it is designed to be before you choose.

* * *

When I started, I didn't use directions because Frank Jones didn't work like that. Frank's main focus was inhibition. Then I started practicing direction, experimenting with bending, going into sitting, and coming to standing, while using several mirrors placed at angles so I could see myself from the side. I did so for years.

* * *

When you start to give directions, register the intention and then stop. Thoughts can also become habitual. We want to stay as close to the nervous system as possible, with intention. So when you give directions, register the intention and then stop, listen, and see what happens.

* * *

My focus on intention began when I was a serious runner. I began running seriously in Santa Barbara, California while in graduate school working for a doctoral degree. For two years, from 1970-72, I ran along the beach on the University of California campus. I continued running after moving to Boston in 1972 to take up a faculty position at Tufts University, and maintained my running schedule until 2003 when my wife died and I had sole responsibility for both my children. On one run in 1973 along the banks of the Charles River, which separates Boston from Cambridge, I decided to give directions while running. I would cease my run and walk for a bit, then run again. And I noticed that once I began to walk and give the primary directions, even before I could actually give them, their effect was already noted. My intention was sufficient and I concluded that because my entire system had been activated by my running, it needed very little encouragement from my thought process.

On "The Arms Support the Back"

We are always integrated. However, the degree of integration can be compromised, and we can behave as if we are not integrated. The purpose of the Alexander work is to come to a realization of when we are behaving as if we are not integrated, and then behave otherwise.

You can't isolate your integration within yourself. On the contrary, you are always integrated relative to what you are doing, what you are thinking, and your environment.

The prevalent way of thinking is to view the back as supporting the arms. That goes along with a focus on doing, on not acknowledging support in being, on adjusting and managing the moment. If you only focus on what you are doing — say, gripping the steering wheel, etc. — that will be your experience. The back will support the movement. But, if at the same time you are aware of the integration of the being supporting the doing, suddenly it isn't just one direction (that of the back supporting the arms). Rather, the arms are also providing input for the whole system, and supporting your back.

We are always reaching out for things. We favor moving forward — doing — at the expense of being. The idea is to touch someone while still staying in your support. Alexander called this "the arms support the back."

On Monkey

Alexander's pupils came up with the term "monkey" to describe the innate bending at hips, knees, and ankles that all primates do, including ourselves — think of how young children bend in their legs without also bending in their lower backs the way so many adults do. Alexander viewed monkey as "a position of mechanical advantage" whether it was a slight bend from uprightness or anywhere in-between to a deep squat. I think of it as a relative position of tensegritive advantage. Going into monkey makes your own system dynamic, it gives you a sense of being in support because you are spring-loaded. When you go into monkey while placing your hands on a person, you call on your own being in support.

* * *

Q. Do you teach monkey to private students?

A. Not usually. I favor bringing the work to the person in the life they lead — rather than bringing the person to the work.

I do explain how we are each comprised of an organized system which developed over unfathomable millions of years of evolution, from the sea to quadruped to biped. I explain the chair work, which Frank Pierce Jones termed "sit-to-stand work." I demonstrate sit-to-stand and show how prevalent it is to engage in some version of the following pattern: dorsiflexing the head — thereby unnecessarily throwing the head and neck muscles, especially the trapezius and the sternocleidomastoid muscles, into tensional imbalance — which then pulls the head closer to the body, pushes your shoulders forward, and depresses the larynx. Then I explain how this tendency is largely habitual, and when inhibited allows the head to move more freely at the atlanto-occipital joint and consequently affect the total pattern of neuromuscular, skeletal, and fascial movement throughout the body. This demonstration is usually confined to a few minutes. Then I demonstrate how specific activities involve the movement associated with monkey or sit-to-stand. Since I live in the Boston area, and my studios have always been in Cambridge, I have always had my share of students who are scientists and medical people. When working with them, I seldom use the term monkey. When I do use the term monkey, I describe rooms in their homes that call for varying versions of monkey. The kitchen, for instance, often occasions the movement associated with monkey (full upright to deep squat) as we access a pot or pan stored in a lower cabinet.

*   *   *

Monkey is a really good way of integrating the nervous system, the being and the doing.

*   *   *

Monkey is aligning yourself relative to what you want to do in the most tensegritive, integrated way possible. Monkey stimulates the tensegritive aspect of the self.

*   *   *

Monkey is a state of mind, open and dynamic.

*   *   *

Monkey is any position where you are in dynamic balance relative to what you are doing.

*   *   *

When you move into bending from full upright toward a squat (or in Alexander parlance, "go into monkey"), you have the potential to reorganize yourself in a way that lets you find the most appropriate usage in relation to what you are doing: meeting yourself being yourself.

On the Moment as a Movement

The moment is a movement
The present is your choice to belong to that moment
And go wherever the road takes you
Change takes place in the ongoing present
And its movement wherever the road takes you

And all change takes place in the ongoing present in
the space between things
Between inhalation and exhalation
Between sunrise and sunset
Between stimulus and response
Between and in the midst of all one chooses to belong
to, whether it be your choice
Or whether in the soft beacon of awareness you
simply discover you are there, right where and how
you knew you belonged.

Questions and Answers

Q: What does it mean to be really present?

A: What in the dickens does it mean to be present anyway? First of all, your body is present. However, when you are not consciously embodied, you are not fully present. When you acknowledge relationship, you move towards the present. When you are out of relationship, you are not present. And again being present is your choice to belong fully to a given moment.

The moment, like the ongoing present, is a movement. And the present is your choice to belong to that movement and to go where the road takes you. Subsequent change takes place between stimulus and response, and whatever choices you make are occasioned by your belonging to the moment.

You become aware of a moment as it begins to surface. Usually, almost as soon as you become aware of the present, it is already changing into the next present moment. This is why I speak of becoming aware of the present surfacing. If, while looking across a room at a social gathering, your attention was drawn to a particular person and you wished to explore more about them and you felt that person might also feel the same from having exchanged glances and if you chose to allow each succeeding present moment to surface exactly as it is, then you would truly find out where that interaction may take you. Perhaps it would lead to an actual dialog between you. Staying present as the road unfolds moment to moment would give each of you a sense of mutual belonging in the moment. What takes you out of being present is reaction, for example trying to get to the relationship you want even if that is not what turns out to be surfacing.

You have a little bit more time than you think. On your way between here and where you are going next, you are usually thinking about where you are going. If instead you think about, "This is me having this experience of walking," you will be more present, time slows down.

Once a Harvard minister questioned one of my trainee teachers about what it meant to be embodied and asked her how could he embody his faith. She invited him to visit our training course. When he came to the training, I asked him what he would do to express his faith. He answered "I would pray." "And how would you pray?" I asked. "I would sit here on this cushion." "Okay," I replied, "have a seat, and so you don't feel conspicuous to the rest of the group I will ask everyone to sit in a circle and join you." To the group I suggested they might pray if they wished, meditate or just sit in a quiet silence of thought. Everyone sat in the circle and while the minister was praying I put hands on his head, neck back, shoulders, and forehead, coming back and forth with one emphasis after another to embody his thought, his prayer. After about fifteen minutes I asked, "What was your experience?" He claimed that he probably had for the first time a fully embodied sense of prayer and he then asked whether I would give a talk on embodying faith to all his graduate students in ministry at Harvard. And so I did.

* * *

Q: When you work with a person, are you trying to put them in a particular posture?

A: You aren't trying to change a person's posture. You are trying to help them create awareness of what they are doing to create a posture. You diffuse the neuromuscular pattern, but also work with the person's commitment to holding an idea of who she thinks she needs to be. You do not have an end in sight. You do have a vision of what happens when anyone is not committed to a particular way of being. A person's commitment to being who they think they need to be shows up as a neuromuscular pattern.

Everyone's commitment to habit is different. If you find a way to commit to being yourself, it will inevitably find expression in the relationship of the head/neck.

In working with a person, first and foremost you need to introduce freedom within the existing structure. Instead of imposing something — giving someone a new posture — you need to give the person a chance to experience being free where they are.

You must put your hands on who the person is, not who you want them to be. Give them the experience of being free. It may be emotional, joyful, or sad.

* * *

Q: How do I keep the feeling I get from an Alexander lesson after the lesson has finished? How do I do it on my own?

A: People are always asking me some version of the following: "When I leave your studio, I feel great! I want to keep this feeling. But my new experience fades and I gradually revert to how I was before. How do I learn to find this experience again on my own?"

The answer of course, is not to try to find what no longer exists except vividly in your memory (i.e. your new experience of being you). No experience is meant to last. What endures is your awareness of potential (from the new experience in being you) apart from the probable (from the accustomed experience in being you). But how do we explain this so that they will readily understand, and how do we teach so as to emphasize awareness born from the experience?

What if I were to provide you with an answer along the lines of: "When I am working with you verbally or through touch, you have a different awareness of potential in being you apart from your accustomed behavior, and that lets you have a different experience. When I take my hands away, I promise to leave you with your new awareness born from your new experience. You own that. It is more enduring than the physical changes that are a part of your new experience. You have learned something, and from this learning you have a deeper insight and understanding of you, of who you are or might become should you choose potential over familiarity. Inherent in any meaningful experience lies an exploration of awareness born from the new experience you just had as a means of making lasting changes."

And another answer is: instead of trying to keep what you have gotten from an Alexander lesson, just give it away. Share with someone else the way that you have been communicated with. Focus on your insight derived from the experience.

When a student asks how they can find integration on their own, ask them what they were up to in their thinking as the habit re-asserts itself. For example, consider singing. As you do, can you feel kinesthetically the postural set? You have to practice awareness over and over. Catch yourself in your habit and withhold definition. Give yourself the time.

*   *   *

Q: As a student, the teacher shows me how to feel integrated. The moment after that, I'm trying to think in my brain about how to hold onto it and keep my head positioned.

A: That is about your allegiance to who you think you are. The teacher provides you with a slight window between stimulus and response, between doing and being. It takes a long time to let go of habit and take in new and more valuable information.

The student who experienced the full integration is the same person who had the various issues and conditions before. You have to let go of who you think you have to be. It's about the use of the *self*. The self can't be separated from the body. You are designed to process all these experiences, especially if you work closer to the way you are designed to work.

Aphorisms

Notice when in your thinking you think you know what will happen. Then you miss all the other possibilities.

* * *

If a person is tense, often the only way she will be aware of the tension is when she experiences its absence.

* * *

My deepest moments of change have been when I let myself see something for how it is or seems to be and let myself be moved by it, without trying to do anything.

* * *

You can't not have an embodied experience, but you can behave as if you are not embodied.

* * *

A lesson should be a celebration of each person being alive.

* * *

What is freeing the neck, really? It is simply not continuing to do what you are accustomed to do, and in that moment, the organism will show up in the way it is designed to work.

* * *

If you don't let yourself live through the experience you are actually having, you tend to invite a similar experience again and again. The brain isn't particularly fond of leftovers.

* * *

The less inclined you are to manage your experience, the more you are able to take in, and you are more available to what is around you. That will tend to take you out of the head-forward, pulled down state.

* * *

For me, the only real valid reason for changing yourself is to be more present for the person in front of you.

* * *

The ultimate use of self is to make peace with yourself.

* * *

Do you wish to be seen as an Alexander teacher or for who you are?

* * *

If you've done the best you can, then the result is the best you can get at this moment.

* * *

You can't be heard until you're listened to.

*   *   *

Some days are easy… today is Someday.

*   *   *

Change can take place in a moment of genuine awakening, or gradually over time in a compilation of moments.

*   *   *

Make peace with yourself so you can be at peace with yourself.

*   *   *

What we exercise in the Alexander practice is the practical application of kinesthetic awareness.

*   *   *

The closer you get the farther away you are.

*   *   *

I teach consciousness and its practical application to life.

*   *   *

I will never try to know you, I will always long to see you.

There is no beginning… there is no end…

Some time after my wife Julie died, I traveled to Santa Barbara to spread her ashes in the ocean near where we had spent our first two years living together. When we lived there, you would walk through a eucalyptus grove, then wildflowers, then sand dunes, and finally onto the beach where you stood before the vast and beautiful Pacific ocean. Now it is a nature preserve, with a guard, and you are not allowed on the beach. But I go onto the beach, and tell the guard I want to spread my wife's ashes. The guard is a young student, and he doesn't know what to do, so he says OK.

I stand there, at the water's edge, my bare feet in the wet space between sand and ocean. The tide comes in. My feet sink slightly into the wet sand. I drop ashes. They are taken out to sea, small golden flakes of previous existence drawn quickly back into the ocean. The tide returns as quickly and I drop more ashes into the still point between coming and going. I do this several times. Then there is a soft interruption to my thoughts. Julie becomes present in my thoughts. "I came in with the tide, I left with the tide. There is no beginning, there is no end. I'll return with the tide… and so will you. There is no beginning… there is no end…"

Acknowledgments

_____

I am immensely grateful to all who contributed to this book to ensure its manifestation. And to be clear, I didn't write this book. I spoke this book. Teaching in the abstract is a wonderful skill, but one I don't have in great measure. I find I teach best when working with a specific person or group, responding to their particular needs and questions. In this situation, the teaching emerges through the interaction between us. It is, therefore, especially important to me to acknowledge and thank the students, colleagues, and friends who have, in one way or another, been my teachers over the years. Please forgive me if I have managed to misspell any of your names — it does not in any way diminish my debt to you.

Without Rachel Prabhakar's encouragement, persistence, and devotion we would never have transformed a graduation gift into a book meant for the public. Her desire to make me readable was matched by her editorial skill and singular depth of insight along the way. For her perseverance in bringing this book to fruition I am grateful.

To have the assistance of the brilliant hand and mind of my long time friend and colleague, David Gorman, was a tremendous gift. David designed the book's covers and layout, provided thoughtful suggestions and comments, corrected typos, and guided me through the publication process. Without David and Rachel as a team, this book would not exist.

And to the members of my teacher training courses throughout the years since 1983, grateful thanks for reading what you've heard dozens of times already. To my two principal teaching assistants, Debi Adams and Bob Lada, who have been with me in the training for nearly thirty years, I thank you both for all your years of commitment and dedication. I am grateful to Debi for reading the earliest manuscript and contributing her touching and heartfelt Introduction, and to Bob for his circumspect eye as to what is most appropriate in communication.

To the many students and colleagues who contributed to the specificity of this book through the past 44 years of teaching, I am blessed by our encounter. To Corinne Cassini, who reminded me of who I am, to Caroline Poppink for reminding me of who she was and how change is a delicate balance, to Eileen Troberman for encouraging me to write, to Maya Dolder for reminding me I teach my vision, to Doris Dietschy for appreciating innovation, to Julian Lage for giving me the experience of articulating who I was touching, to Jamee Culbertson, for all her years of care and support, to Angela Leidig for growing beyond her expectations, to Paloma Salud López for appreciating who she is, to Betsy Polatin for asking me to start a teacher training course, which unwittingly transformed my life, hers, and others through her own teaching, to Anna Tolstoy for finding her calling, to Jennifer Roig-Francoli for discovering freedom is her birthright. To playwright, Tennessee Williams for introducing me to key lime pie over illuminating life-changing lunch conversations. To Ursula Zidek for keeping it all together through thick and thin times! To Rosa Luisa Rossi who introduced me to Michelangelo's sculpture of 'David' embodying 'Inhibition as direct experience'. To film actor and producer, Michael Douglas for his generosity of spirit, always. To John Arvanties who insisted I break barriers to which I complied. To Eiji Tanamura and Toru Matsushima for their counsel, hospitality, and friendship. To Andrea Studer and Priska Schelbert-Gauger for their years of commitment to study and for their beautiful families and for so many years of friendship. To Spencer Schaefer for teaching me simplicity of approach in matters complex. To Sophie Wolf and Pierre Lauper for cherished years together. To Eva Wirth and Simon for all your care and hospitality. To Pippa Bondy for finding her way. To Manuelle Bogel for her commitment to life long study. To Martin Weinkle for his appreciation for the preservation of the enduring value of the written word. To Christine Robb in appreciation for illuminating insights given freely for so many years. To Scott Zeigler, then Artistic Director of the Institute for Advanced Theater Training, American Repertory Theater at Harvard University and now Dean of the North Carolina School for the Arts, for hiring me to teach the graduate acting students who were golden throughout my twelve years at Harvard. How wonderful to be reminded how much I love working with actors. I hope that all of you who were in the Institute for

Advanced Theater Training and whose individual names are too numerous to list, learned as much from me as I was privileged to learn from you.

And a special heartfelt thanks to my perpetual teachers for all they have taught me; my adult children, Adrianna, Danielle, and Gabriel.

I also wish to thank the following people for consistently hosting workshops, serving as translators, and for contributing to this book in some meaningful way: Marie-Françoise le Foll and Eillen Sellam for launching my teaching in Europe in 1988 after the first International Congress for Alexander teachers in 1986 which has set in motion all the workshops, David Gorman for helping me become known in the UK by inviting me to teach regularly in his London training course, and Alan Rosenberg (coach for the USA Olympic Rowing Crew) and Stanley Rosenberg for their invitation to serve as special assistant to the Rowing Crew.

Also thanks (in alphabetical order) to Ann Seelye, Annie Turner, Annie Weinkle, Anthony Kingsley, Arnaud Grelier, Barbara Paton, Betsy Hestnes, Caroline Chalk, Celia Jurdant-Davis, Chris Friedman, Constance Clare-Newman, Damian Köppel, Daria Okugawa, Dr. David Griesemer, Diana Bradley, Diana Glenn, Dominique Depuis, Ellen Bierhorst, Elyse Shafarman, Fritz Papst, Gabriele Breuninger, Galit Ziff, Gilles Estran, Glenna Batson, Graham Elliott, Greg Marposon, Hillary White, Holly Cinnamon, Hubert Goddard, Isabelle Augustin, Jeremy Chance, Jessica Webb, Joan Fitzgerald, Joseph and Maria Weiss, Kanae Tsuneki, Kate Howe, Kathleen Morrison, Kathryn Amour, Kay Kim, Ken Anno, Ken Thompson, Malcom Balk, Manuelle Borgel, Margrit Gysin, Mariela Cárdonas, Matthias Schelbert, Mayumi Shimizu, Meike Dubbert, Melissa Matson, Michael Frederick, Michael Gelb, Michiel Poppink, Mike Serio, Monika Kopp, Naoko Matsushiro, Nial Kelly, Olivia Rohr, Patricia Kuypers, Patricia O'Neil, Paul and Tessa Versteeg, Penny O'Conner, Philippe Cotton, Priscilla Endicot, Rebecca Gwynn-Jones, Renate Wehner, Richard Brennan, Richard Ortner, Rivka Cohen, Robin Eastham, Sabine Grosser, Sakiko Ishitsubo, Sara Solnik, Seong-un Kim, Serina Bardola, Shigeko Suzuki, Sooyeon Kim, Stephane Ryder, Tine Gherardi, Wendy Cook, Yasuhiro Ishida, Yuriko Ishii, my current training course members: Anita Freeman, Brian Griffen, Diane Sales, Jan Muller, Kremenia Stephaniva, Martha Juelich, Michelle Lemp, Miriam Bolkosky, Nicole Kootz, Ruth Libbey, Sarah Bond, thank you all. To Mary Jonaitas and Michael, to Kurt Leland and Charles for encompassing perspective. To Rikka Cohen, Yuzuru Katagiri, Elisabeth Walker, Bill Walsh, and to all the people throughout so many years of teaching who have in their own ways contributed to this book. I cannot list you all, however you know who you are.

And a special thanks to Neal Katz, for suggesting the book's title, *Touching Presence*, during a brief and unexpected encounter and conversation on my way to my studio early one morning. Without this encounter I might very well have chosen *Touching Beauty*. Now I think *Touching Presence* best reflects the essence of the book, for in any encounter with another person before they speak and before they act, before they give you indication through word and action who they are, you are moved simply by the presence of their being.

To Elisabeth Schanda who in May of this year in Linz, Austria provided quiet space in her apartment and in her being for me to assemble my ideas for the manuscript far away from my consuming life in Cambridge, Massachusetts. I'm grateful, Elisabeth, for your love throughout our years together and especially when most needed to complete the book.

And lastly, posthumously to Dr. Frank Pierce Jones, my colleague, mentor, and friend, for seeing something in an angry young man. Your teaching changed my life.

Thank you all.

Tommy Thompson,
Cambridge, Massachusetts
August 2019

About Tommy Thompson

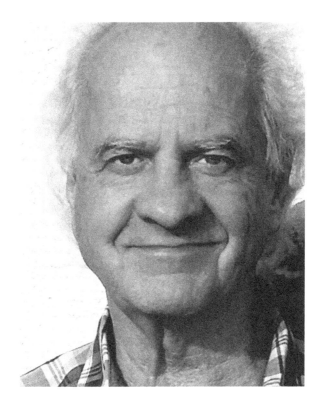

Since 1975 Tommy Thompson has taught the Alexander Technique to professional and Olympic athletes, dressage riders, musicians, dancers, actors, scientists, physicians, corporate and university professionals, children, and the disabled. He has an active private teaching practice and has given over 900 workshops for Alexander teachers, teacher trainees and the general public in the USA, Canada, Ireland, England, France, Spain, the Netherlands,

Switzerland, Germany, Austria, Italy, Hungary, Israel, Japan, and Korea. Tommy is Founder and Director of the Alexander Technique Center at Cambridge, which has been training Alexander Technique teachers since 1983. He served as special assistant to the 1976 Olympic USA Heavyweight Rowing Crew.

He was on the faculty at Harvard University for 12 years where he taught the Technique to graduate students enrolled in the American Repertory Theater/Moscow Art Theater School Institute for Advanced Theater Training. A former Assistant Professor of Drama and Managing Director of Tufts Arena Theater at Tufts University, Tommy has acted in or directed over 200 theater productions, working with such notable artists as Jerzy Grotowski, Michael Douglas, Jerry Turner, Georgi Paro, Robert E. Lee and with Tennessee Williams in a revival of *Eccentricities of a Nightingale* (1977).

Tommy is co-founder, charter member, and was first Chair of Alexander Technique International (ATI). His contributions to ATI earned him the ATI Lifetime Membership Award. He is also an Honorary Member of ATI France (ATIF), the Irish Society of Alexander Technique Teachers (ISATT), and a teaching member of the Japan Alexander Technique Association (JATA).

He also co-founded the Alexander Technique Association of New England (ATA) in 1982 and the Frank Pierce Jones Archives and the F. Matthias Alexander Archives, initially housed in the Wessell Library at Tufts University. He was ATA's director for six years.

Tommy is co-author of *Scientific and Humanistic Contributions of Frank Pierce Jones*, and has contributed numerous papers on the Alexander work, Tai Chi, and theater to Alexander and theater journals, periodicals, martial arts journals, and newsletters. Tommy has taught in over thirty teacher-training courses around the world, presented papers at both the First and Second International Congresses for Alexander Teachers, was one of the Second Generation Teachers invited to give master classes at the Third International Congress and has consistently given Continuous Learning classes at the congresses since their inception.

Tommy is currently writing a novel, *Just Like Always*, while beginning another book on the Alexander work.

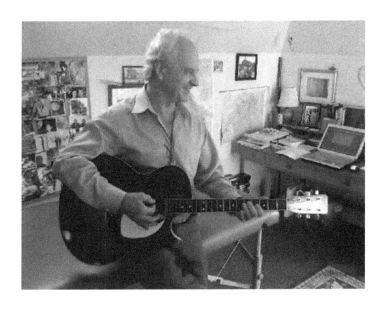

About Rachel Prabhakar

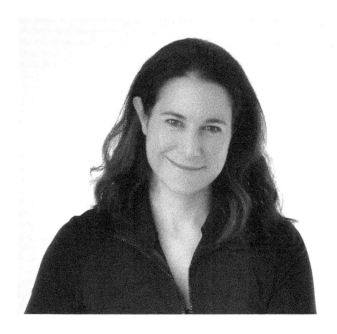

Rachel Prabhakar teaches the Alexander Technique and Pilates at her metro Boston studio, and Pilates at Boston University. Her practice serves people with a wide variety of medical conditions and injuries, as well as dancers and athletes.

In addition to teaching private students and groups, Rachel has conducted a variety of workshops, including employee wellness programs at Boston University and the Boston Museum of Fine Arts, Pilates teacher trainings, and workshops for adult ballet students. She has also worked with injured dance students at the Boston Conservatory.

Rachel trained with Tommy Thompson at the Alexander Technique Center at Cambridge and with Debi Adams at the Boston Conservatory, graduating in 2013 and receiving ATI sponsorship in 2014. She went on to complete further post-graduate work with Tommy Thompson.

Rachel received her Pilates Level 2 Instructor certification from the Australian Pilates Method Association (APMA) in 2009, and then completed an advanced apprenticeship at the renowned Melbourne studio, Balance & Control. Prior to undertaking Pilates certification, Rachel spent a decade working as a software engineer. She holds a BA from Cornell University and an MA from the University of Chicago.

Rachel lives in Brookline, MA, USA with her husband and two daughters.

Articles by Tommy Thompson & Others

Articles about the Alexander Technique are available on Tommy's website, at www.easeofbeing.com/articles. As of this printing, the following articles are available on the website:

At the Heart of Teaching or 'A Brilliant Disguise'

Keynote Address given at the 2nd International Alexander Teachers' Conference, Dublin, Ireland, 2017

Sun and Moon

Talk given at the 6th International Congress of the Alexander Technique, Freiburg, Germany, 1999, on the day of the eclipse of the sun by the moon.

Moving from the Still Point of Support: An Interpretation of the Alexander Technique

(*also available in Japanese translation*)

Anam Cara

Keynote Address delivered at the Alexander Technique International Annual General Meeting, Spanish Point, Ireland, 2000

The Teaching of Frank Pierce Jones:
   A Personal Memoir

Frank Pierce Jones's Views on the Alexander Technique:
   The moral and humanistic implications of the
   Alexander Technique

Learning How to Learn:
   My Work with the 1976 Olympic Rowing Team

Showing Up

Instructions given to the actors in the American
Repertory Theater / Moscow Art Theater School,
Institute for Advanced Theater Training at Harvard
University about preparing for each class.

(*also available in Japanese translation*)

Making Peace with Yourself is the Ultimate Use of
the Self

Excerpt from Alexander Technique International's
Exchange Journal, Fall 2010

Harvard Women's Health Watch –
Alexander Technique and Chronic Back Pain

Digging Deeper: The Diving-Board Effect

By Julian Lage — Julian trained and qualified as an
Alexander teacher in Tommy Thompson's Training.
Julian also studied with Debi Adams, and later,
with David Gorman.

The Alexander Technique Center at Cambridge

The Alexander Technique Center at Cambridge offers an internationally recognized Teacher Training Program. Founded by Tommy Thompson in 1983 in Cambridge, Massachusetts, the program offers a three-year, 1600-hour course of study.

Upon successfully completing the program and fulfilling all program requirements, graduates receive a Certificate of Qualification in the Alexander Technique.

Each graduate is eligible to become a Certified Teaching Member of Alexander Technique International (ATI), an international professional society of Alexander teachers.

For more information, visit www.easeofbeing.com.

*   *   *

Tommy is available to teach Postgraduate Alexander Technique courses worldwide. For inquiries please write to him at <tommy@easeofbeing.com>.

EaseofBeing Publications™

Touching Presence

Designed by *David Gorman*
Layout and typesetting in *InDesign CS6*
Chapter Titles in 16 pt. *Berlin Sans FB*
Body Text in 13 pt. *Adobe Garamond Pro*
Published and distributed by *EaseofBeing Publications*

CPSIA information can be obtained
at www.ICGtesting.com
Printed in the USA
JSHW021030091019
1862JS00004B/14